Copy for ~~Patricia~~

D1121699

THE CHILDREN'S HOUR:

A LIFE IN CHILD PSYCHIATRY

ALSO BY KENNETH S. ROBSON

The Borderline Child: Approaches to Etiology, Diagnosis, and Treatment (1983)

A Great and Glorious Game: Baseball Writings of A. Bartlett Giamatti (1998)

THE CHILDREN'S HOUR:
A LIFE IN CHILD PSYCHIATRY

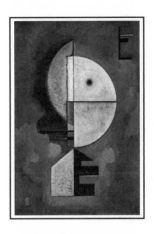

Kenneth S. Robson, M.D.

Lyre Books

West Hartford, Connecticut

Library of Congress Control Number: 2010931260

ISBN: 978-0-615-39198-4

First Edition, 2010

Cover painting by permission:

Vasily Kandinsky
Upward (Empor), October 1929
Oil on cardboard
27 ½ x 19 ¼ inches (70 x 49 cms)
The Solomon R. Guggenheim Foundation,
Peggy Guggenheim Collection, Venice, 1976
76.2553.35

© 2010 Artists Rights Society (ARS), New York / ADAGP, Paris

Author photograph by Lorraine Greenfield

Published by
Lyre Books
West Hartford, Connecticut
lyrebooks@aol.com

To the children and families whose lives have touched mine.
With most I made contact, relieved distress and
provided comfort. For some I helped open
doors to the future. We have
changed one another.
I remember.

Aknowledgements

Lee Rubin-Collins and Robert Lobis were helpful critics of early drafts and later revisions of the manuscript. Joanne Sommers, as always, was an invaluable resource from conception to completion. My best friend and best critic, my wife Bonnie, in her usual gentle way, was an astute editor and, along with my son Sam, an always available booster club when the game was in doubt. And Lenore Terr's final edit was invaluable.

TABLE OF CONTENTS

INTRODUCTION

This book describes the labor I love: my work in the inner sanctums of troubled children and their families. Its passion lasts and its poetry, too. I write to capture, preserve and pass along to new practitioners and interested others the beauty of my years spent playing – for keeps.

The war room of children's lives is a shadowy, well-guarded space. Access may be denied. Entry is a privilege using skills hard won, skills that rely on familiarity with the anatomy of children's souls: rust-free and closer to the surface of being than those of their opaque adult counterparts. Passwords are required, even in desperate circumstances. Breaking and entering only heightens security concerns. The task at hand requires some combination of poet, private investigator, bird-watcher, translator and flim-flam man to establish what is right and strong and sturdy enough to keep or get life moving. It is healthy tissue that is precious – symptoms and signs are often noise, not signal. Development, like the idle of those new hybrid cars, runs silently.

The language of this work is metaphor. We are creatures of symbol. The physician to children's maladies of mind and spirit must be fluent in this language if the cloth is to hold. Dialogue creates the words. In metaphor resides the power of those words. But metaphor is fast becoming a lost tongue, dusty from disuse, unappreciated, even unknown. Freud said it well: "Wherever I go, the poet has been there first."

The history of child psychiatry, like that of childhood itself, is brief. Hardly a century has passed since the discovery that children suffer all of the afflictions of adults as well as disorders specific to the early years of life. In the beginning, biological frames of reference for childhood disorder were primary in Europe. In America, after World War II, the lure of the psychoanalytic model dominated training programs and systems of diagnostic classification into the 1970s, when biological influences began to establish their credibility and psychoanalytic modes fell into disfavor. But without psychoanalytic glue the work is literal, synthetic and two-dimensional. Stripped of its beauty, it lacks authenticity. George Nakashima, the great furniture designer, spent many hours searching for the pieces of wood that would allow him to go with the existing grain, to highlight their intrinsic form. He was wise in his unwillingness to savage nature.

Since the most powerful tool the child psychiatrist possesses is her or himself, this book is also about me. My scalpels and poultices are personal. Their use requires imagination, proper timing and nimble delivery. While we are physicians, we are also choreographers. Our textbooks are the nuances of facial expression, the telltale posture of despair, thought run amok in mania or running on empty in schizophrenia.

I entered child and adolescent psychiatry at a time when the specialty was valued within the medical community and the public eye. Psychoanalysis as a model permeated the best training sites such as the Harvard programs where I trained. My teachers, many of them European émigrés from Nazism, effortlessly combined the art and science of working with children. They knew and appreciated the importance of play, imagination, terror and beauty in the developing spirits of the young. Deeply cultured, they saw life and death at their ugliest as precious and worthy of scrutiny, even when no longer amenable to change. Most of these gifted mentors are now dead; and the burgeoning of scientific psychiatry coupled with the crush of managed care leaves little time to pursue their precious clinical and scientific legacies. *Sic transit gloria mundi.*

Child and adolescent psychiatry is a trade as well as an art and a science. It requires apprenticeships with master craftsmen. To learn a craft in depth requires repetition, reflection, and study of the brilliant pieces of literature painstakingly created only a generation or two ago. These classics rest upon the unchanging, recurrent dilemmas, internal, external and interpersonal, with which every child, past, present or future, struggles. I was schooled in this extraordinary body of work and blessed to learn from many of its authors. I am indebted to them for eliciting from me whatever gifts I have brought to my table. They were my Nakashimas.

My character and temperament are a proper fit for child psychiatry. The mass of mankind, with considerable effort, struggles to leave the early years behind. Aside from a few idealized and distorted recollections, the anxiety, fearful dependence, vulnerability and pain of childhood and adolescence are encumbrances to the business of living. They drop out of awareness. Like an iceberg sinking, only fragments of disconnected, consciously meaningless memory remain floating on the surface of mind. But there are some creative beings, artists of every stripe, who retain ready access to remembrance of their earliest years, traveling backward or forward through time. For a child psychiatrist, his or her childhood is the darkroom that develops time past and time present simultaneously. Time travel, back to the future, comes easily to me.

As a child, I was sensitive to the feelings of others, sometimes in the extreme, too eager to help, loath to hurt. My big-screen radar was both asset and liability when reading, or over-reading, the gestures of human relationships: bodily movement, posture, facial expression, tone of voice. But in my clinical work this same hypersensitivity became a valuable, efficient diagnostic and therapeutic tool. It also filled my world with repeated moments of pleasure, visceral responses to Beauty –

which is, wherever I find it, my religion. My work is filled with many venues where beauty resides: my wife and children, the Boston Red Sox, fishing, boxing, classical music, poetry, fine art, rocks and red-tailed hawks. all these get bit parts or leading roles in my diaolgues with patients and their families.

Over the years I have worked with hundreds of children of all ages, as well as adults whose childhoods are still very much alive, frozen in time by terror, sorrow, loss or illness. While most of these patients have been seen in a clinical context for diagnosis and/or treatment, some have been forensic in nature. That is, they have been referred for evaluation in the context of court actions such as divorce, liability for psychological damages, or criminal charges such as sexual assault or murder. Be their cases clinical or forensic in origin, certain of these patients loom large in my memory. They serve as the text of my career and this book. My involvement with them lasted from a few hours to many years. However lengthy that involvement, contact with these children and their families over the span of life and death has kept me in constant proximity to the natural rhythms and cycles of life, its beauty, its deformations, its tragedies, its triumphs over adversity.

Rather than construct my narrative around typical diagnostic classifications of childhood disorders, which can be two-dimensional and unrelated to life, I have grouped children, and some adults, into thematic collages composed of multiple patients of varying age, sex and manner of presentation. Some are described in depth as central to a theme, while others provide briefer vignettes that amplify and/or elaborate upon the core concern. The chapters of this book are arranged to reflect the progressive phases of normal development. Since my own feelings, reactions, perceptions and strategies are intrinsic to therapeutic success or failure, I have tried to bring the reader close to or even into my experience so that both the style and content of my work, and the patients themselves, take shape once again, come to life from their records, my memories and some current interviews. I hope that the text reflects the depth of my pleasure in working with these children and their families as they illustrate, in the chapters of my life and theirs, this privileged profession's travels and travails through the collected volumes of the human comedy.

The identities of the children and their families herein have been altered to protect their privacy. Otherwise, all of the case material, therapeutic efforts, and outcomes accurately reflect the author's experience.

P ractice an art for love and the happiness of your life. You will find it outlasts almost everything but breath.

– Katherine Anne Porter

THE CHILDREN'S HOUR:

A LIFE IN CHILD PSYCHIATRY

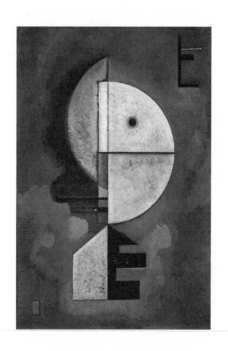

CHAPTER ONE: HYSTERIA

What is our life? A play of passion,
Our mirth the music of division:
Our mother's wombs the tiring houses be
Where we are dressed for this short comedy.

– Sir Walter Raleigh

The pelvis is our skeletal center of gravity, the hub of our upright world. It bears the torso's weight from above and the relentless pounding of locomotion from below. Its several bones are joined into a kettle-like structure with a narrow, ovoid outlet that forms the birth canal. Within the pelvic cavity rest vital organs, among them the tools of procreation. In women, over the course of pregnancy, the pelvic joints give way, softening and stretching to accommodate the occupancy and exit of their *locum tenens* boarder. When push comes to shove, nature defers to youth.

In parallel fashion, the map of mind, resistant to any change in its established boundaries, bows to the brash demands for space laid down by the impatient Johnny-come-lately who arrives prepared to take up rent-free residence. Experienced clinicians know, from psychological test data gathered during pregnancy, that mind, like pelvis, bends only at a price. Gestation and insanity yield virtually indistinguishable test profiles. Madness and pregnancy are cut from the same pattern but different cloth. The fluidity of the mental apparatus seen in psychosis results from compound fractures of essential structures. In pregnancy those structures remain intact but acquire a benign and temporary state of plasticity that can mimic the disordered thought and psychic looseness seen in grave deterioration of mind.

During pregnancy the self, in its attempts to incorporate a new and unfamiliar other, exhibits bizarre appetites, primitive fears, morbid preoccupations and volcanic eruptions. There is merit in the ancient Greek notion that hysteria results when an unquiet uterus looses its moorings and wanders aimlessly about the pelvic cavity in a peripatetic search for home. It is no wonder that pregnancy's darker sides speak the language of Molly Bloom's soliloquy in Joyce's *Ulysses* and keen with the mournful, otherworldly echoes of the whale.

Cleo, an olive-skinned mother of four, found herself pregnant again. Pacing the floors of her Beacon Hill townhouse, this caustic, diminutive Boston beauty railed against her state, raging at father and fetus alike. Her lamentations were recorded in a Joycean narrative she dropped casually in my lap as her opening statement, before seating herself at our initial meeting. Such documents are often like the opening notes of a symphony. What follows are variations on that theme. Cleo was referred by a former patient of mine who had witnessed with mounting alarm the erratic turns of mood and near-miss collisions resulting from her friend's gestational turmoil. Cleo speaks from the heart and from her wandering womb:

"I seemed to be in a dark mood...until I got home...there was no toilet paper...I started screaming, I frighten everyone...could have killed myself...I cried and ate a bowl of ice cream just like a fat person would do. I hate fat people; they have no self-control, neither do I. Can't get my fat ass going in the morning. Stacks of life are piling up around me. I just want to swim. I don't feel heavy in water. People tell me I'm getting big. I guess it is real. There is something, a boy inside me. Will some maternal instinct kick in? He wants to name it Micah; too biblical for my taste. I just don't

care much what it is called. Something bad will happen because of all these bad thoughts.

"I couldn't swim last night due to Martin Luther King. What the hell kind of holiday is that anyway? I am having somewhat clear thoughts of today, must be all the sugar. I remember quite vividly all of my violent thoughts for the past six months. I should have thrown that ugly necklace at him he gave me...stones of blue dug out of the ground. I am not a heavy stone person. 'Pearls,' asshole, 'I said I like pearls.' Could it be I don't tolerate men very well? Good thing my thoughts don't transpire into events.

"I hate everything. I dreamt of my grandmother. I kept looking and couldn't find her. I realized she was dead. I forgot. Last week I dreamt I climbed up a steep, slippery, ice-covered mountain with my father. I was wearing my wedding dress. I was surprised it still fit as my stomach had gotten so fat. I started sliding down...concerned the dress would get dirty...there were steep rocks and a drop into space. I kept wondering why the rocks weren't hurting me as my body tossed into them. It appears I am having a kid, I also dreamt of that for the first time last night (besides having a miscarriage) I wouldn't look at it when it was born though. Looks should mean nothing. I should be praying for a healthy child. Didn't I receive enough from my mother? She was in the dream last night, yelling at me for my behavior toward the kid. I think I got up and left the hospital swearing that the floors were dirty and I was going for a swim. I'd be back to inspect the kid when I got my head in order. Then, to piss off my mother, I said I'm contemplating putting it up for adoption. Could I? I dabble with the thought. Can I love this kid? Is normal ever going to be real for me? I hate everything today. I won't have to contemplate suicide, this pregnancy will surely kill me.

"I don't think this kid likes me, he senses my feelings. He kicks the shit out of me. I will truly be afraid to look at him when he is

born. This kid is mine. I probably can't give him away no matter what. My demons are back. I can't take care of a baby by myself. He is starting to be real but I hate the feel of fat on my body. Horrible dreams last night: I had the kid, went to look at him... he and other babies not moving, kind of frozen in jars...couldn't find mine, someone stole him. I never had a chance to see him."

Cleo's monologue portrays the more primitive and extreme dislocations of pregnancy: intense ambivalence, infanticide, magical thinking, profound doubts, lost freedom, changing body image, turmoil, deprivation and unfinished family matters revisited and reworked in dreams or nightmares. She longs to swim in amniotic fluid like her unborn son. Such disorganization is a precursor to the advent of a new edifice creating new living space. Regression that precedes developmental progress remains a fundamental law through all stages of the life cycle. Two steps back then three steps forward. Like Wagner's music, the mind in pregnancy sounds worse than it is.

I saw Cleo only a few times prior to the birth of her son Michael. While given to melodrama and hyperbole, she was not a fundamentally troubled person, and I chose to emphasize the adaptive aspects of her mental pandemonium to let her welcome her new arrival in a more receptive frame of mind. She soon fell in love with her son—joy became her portion.

Michael was a beautiful infant who nursed vigorously for eighteen months. He was weaned grudgingly into life as a curious, competent, amusing boy whose charm wore well. Despite family turbulence he grew into a richly endowed, urbane adolescent, though with a mordant take on the world. When I saw him last, at fifteen, he continued to convey the impression that his mother had been, and continued to be, the primary provider of the lovingly prepared sustenance at his table. Just as the pelvic joints, post-partum, return to their normal state of immobility, the jagged edges of psyche are rounded to a kinder, gentler whole greater than the sum of its previous parts. After delivery the turmoil of pregnancy fades into the numbness of memory, much as the pain of childbirth itself is lost to conscious recall like a blurred but precious photograph.

A madwoman's pregnancy is another matter. Maureen embarrassed her tightly wrapped, accountant husband with her crude, sexualized humor, loud voice and endless, flamboyant flirtations. At eighteen, her green eyes and copper hair framed a pale, alabaster face that distracted one from her essential oddness. Her behaviors were regularly forty-five degrees off center, leading onlookers to wince with a discomfort they could not quite articulate. Her husband, in a state of chronic befuddlement, could never gain ground on his frenetic partner as he pursued her in an antic chase through the cluttered corridors of her life. Then, for the first time, Maureen became pregnant. Her restless womb launched cannonades out of the garish underworld of her madness.

Maureen had been under my care for several years prior to her pregnancy with Siobhan. I had seen her through two hospitalizations prompted by psychotic regressions that exhibited delusions and hallucinations. Her mental state at those times, and her family history of disturbance, led to an unfortunate prognosis. She suffered from schizoaffective disorder, a serious and life-long vulnerability that is characterized by periods of uneasy calm punctuated by episodes of total, psychic dissolution. Medications are of great benefit but during pregnancy, especially the first trimester, they put the fetus at risk for certain birth defects .

Because of this risk I opted, after discussing the matter with Maureen and her husband, to take her off all psychotropic agents until she had passed the first trimester without incident.

As her dreams deteriorated into ghoulish scenes of mayhem, I knew that she would soon break the fragile bonds of her sanity and descend into florid psychosis. Dreams are the harbingers of impending madness. She reported nightmares of deformed babies that seemed to talk and act like adults. Repeatedly she dreamed of burying stillborn children and hallucinated the voice of her infant calling out to her after she woke. She ruminated on suicide and went so far as to fashion a noose for herself. I was forced to hospitalize her out of concern for two lives.

Her husband, who badly wanted something good and whole in his fractured life, wondered if good fortune would ever be his lot. As Maureen sank in and out of lunacy, she kept her comic slant on things, allowing both of us to laugh. But the relief was brief. Ruminations that for Cleo remained primarily internal, erupted into all the corners of Maureen's world: her marriage, her family, and her friends. Conception had been painless; conceiving of herself as mother was driving her crazy. Her own mother seemed to have been limited, running out of energy to parent Maureen, who was the youngest of four. To complicate matters, as the gates of her mind swung open, Maureen recalled and dreamt of her mother sexually molesting her in childhood, manually providing enemas and "merry times" by digitally penetrating anus and vagina. Her past provided no resources for her maternal role to call upon and make her own. And in a Catholic family abortion and giving up a child for adoption were out of the question.

Placed again on medications, Maureen careened through the remaining months of her gestation and finally delivered, loudly, a pale girl child who looked somehow fragile. I have, over the years, come to use skin color and turgor as clinical signs of psychological stamina. Siobhan failed my test and entered the world with too little color, vigor and resilience. Maureen now came to our meetings with her rumpled baby and fragmenting life in tow. Like those of some new parents, her movements were awkward. I had been through two infants of my own recently enough to step into the breach with her baby on my lap. Siobhan was not easily soothed by her mother's clumsy efforts. Like her father, she often wore a look of uncertainty, confusion or, sometimes, fear. During one such session Siobhan wailed with increasing intensity until Maureen, overwhelmed, seemingly helpless and on the cusp of murderous rage, rose to her feet and handed her daughter off for safe-keeping. Bolting out the office door, she rushed headlong down the stairs, exiting to the street, with me in hot pursuit. She was found by the police, cowering under a bush, and hospitalized. A frightened Siobhan was retrieved by her father.

This dramatic turn of events propelled Maureen's mother-in-law into action. She moved into her granddaughter's home *in loco parentis.* She was a mature woman and an experienced mother of three whom fortune delivered at the right moment. I continued to follow Maureen and had many occasions to watch her with Siobhan. Her native discomfort with the physical and psychological aspects of parenting persisted. I feared for the future of this chalk-white child who had her mother's red hair and, I hoped, few other traits born of the maternal gene pool.

A fundamental sense in the early months and years of life that the world is unsafe—and for Siobhan this was her reality—can leave the growing child with a profound mistrust of one's self and others that endures throughout life. On the other hand, many children with a deeply troubled parent overcome that adversity and thrive. In similar fashion, five percent of humanity is at genetic risk for schizophrenia, yet only one percent develop the illness. Eighty percent of the vulnerable gene pool is protected by nature, good fortune, and the force of will. In baseball, four for five is an unheard of .800 batting average. One of the great pleasures of my profession is to witness in later life the resilience of children whom one has worried about and managed during their earlier years.

There is another lens through which to regard conception, gestation and birth. Childhood fantasies of pregnancy are a study in their own right. Often they are amusing but demand an attentive audience. My first encounter with such fantasies occurred during my training years when a close friend's jealous three-year-old, now the sister of a new baby, ran screaming into our midst with news that she had just had a baby. "Come and see," she proudly implored, guiding the assembled multitude to the bathroom. There, floating in the toilet, was a fecal stick. "It's a hippo," she cried, "I had a baby hippo." After proper accolades, the newborn was dispensed with in the usual manner, much to the chagrin of the imaginative mother who was forced to witness her offspring flushed out of existence into Boston harbor.

This equating of feces with babies is commonplace and reminds us that, in early childhood, logic takes a back seat to imagination's powerful sway. If you wish it, it is so. The sky's the limit. Anyone can do everything with anything. Sarah, an animated five-year-old, had maternal ambitions similar to most of her peers. Sarah charmed. Her strategic plan, as it emerged in the course of therapy, was singular. Sarah was referred for fears and nightmares, common symptoms in five-year-olds. Atypical in girls was the nightly bed-wetting that infuriated her mother, and embarrassed Sarah who, nonetheless, continued wetting despite her earnest vows of entering a new, dry age.

Sarah loved to draw. She came enthusiastically to her sessions with crayons and paper in hand, ready to spontaneously unravel her troubles in the rainbow hues of Crayola. Her pictures were sunny and full of the life that she herself displayed. Flowers grew in profusion around cozy cottages, dogs and children gamboled about and, always at the center of things, a mother pushed a baby carriage. Though the baby's name changed weekly, the family seemed, in composition, remarkably similar to Sarah's.

Like every responsible homeowner, Sarah was intent on maintaining her gardens through the hot, dry summer. I noticed that watering cans appeared and were used with inordinate glee to flood the beds. "You know, Dr. Robson," she informed me, "flowers don't grow without water; nothing grows without water." I had broken her code. How about babies I inquired innocently. Sarah turned Crayola's deepest shade of red, set down her crayons, and waxed silent. Such abrupt interruptions of play are signposts of anxiety. "Sarah," I commented, "you don't need to water down there for babies to grow. At the right time you'll grow one of your own in your own family in your own house. You'll need to wait until you're ready and that will be soon enough. And," I continued, "if you stop wetting your bed you'll feel more grown up and mom will stop yelling at you." The trade-off apparently felt negotiable; Sarah shortly slept through the night between dry sheets.

When Freud took on the issues of pregnancy and childbirth, from the vantage point of his male-dominated world, he left boys out of the picture, denying them their rightful place in the annals of reproduction. He emphasized the girl's discovery and chagrin over her absent penis and her envy of males for their plumbing. But pregnant parents of boys, if reasonably observant, will catch these virile youngsters pushing out their bellies and pretending they are with child. The extraordinary powers of a mother to grow a new human being do not go unnoticed by male children. False pregnancy and childbirth, *pseudocyesis*, is more common in women but is a well-documented syndrome in males envious of the mysterious feats of mothers and keen to show the world that gender has not undone them. Adam lost a rib that might as well have been a womb.

The anatomy of the ano-genital region is a complicated map for children to master. But add to its orifices, organs, passageways, and products the psychological embellishments of sex, excretory functions and childbirth, with their attendant shame and fascination, and any sensible child must find a simpler way. Conception is easy enough to figure: what goes in the mouth passes to the "stomach" and out of the most familiar hole, the anus. The oral route to pregnancy is a powerful, tenacious fantasy that has been implicated in conditions such as anorexia nervosa and related gastrointestinal syndromes. A seven-year-old girl I evaluated as a victim of alleged sexual abuse had become mute and stopped eating. She had fellated her step-father and was terrified that her wish to have a baby would now, illicitly, be granted. An adolescent honors student referred for evaluation of the sudden onset of panic attacks and a ten-pound weight loss had fellated her boyfriend and shame-facedly wondered with me if she was pregnant. The fantasies of oral impregnation vanquish logic and common sense.

In childhood the fantasy of a cloaca is the rule: one common orifice through which urine, feces, gas, and newborns pass indiscriminately. My three-year-old granddaughter recently asked her mother: "Mom, when I came out how did you keep the pee and poop off of me? How did you get me out of the potty?" The old Jesuit dictum of original sin placed our beginnings where sin properly belongs: *inter urinas et feces*. Since the rectum, for children, is the only familiar orifice out of which anything approaching the weight and mass of an infant may pass, anal birth is logical. Little goes in and less comes out of the vagina, which remains an anatomic mystery to most young children. And texts or illustrations do not correct the anatomic charts of childhood that rest upon what is rather than what might be; feces fall, gas passes and, from that well-lit main exit, with the grace of god, babies, too, enter this world.

The only literary memory of conception that I have found occurs in a wonderful passage at the beginning of Laurence Sterne's *Tristram Shandy,* where Tristram blames his unfortunate life on the fact that his mother interrupted coitus by asking whether a clock had been wound. But similarly bizarre intrusions surface in therapeutic sessions. A depressed patient of mine, the mother of three young children who longed for peace (and sometimes death), dreamed that she was sliding headlong down a spiral tube awash with rusty water. We both wondered if her dream was some old, Bakelite recording of her descent down the birth canal. Be that as it may, familiarity with children's colorful iterations of pregnancy and childbirth is essential if child psychiatrists are to comprehend the tragicomic chapters to come.

The sanitizing process of socialization is a hindrance to effective clinical work with children. The practitioner should be intimately familiar with the mind of the very young child and with his or her own past erotic and excretory experiences. The innocence of childhood is a wish generated by adult anxiety, an editorial about all the news that's unfit to print. I was not a sexually precocious adolescent nor was I naive. But my first pelvic examinations of women in medical school felt illicit. And my initial efforts at catheterization of a female patient could have been a scene showing Laurel and Hardy or Abbott and Costello as medical impostors. As for rectal exams, more often than not I followed the lead of my mentors and wrote in the chart "deferred." When that dodge failed and there was no avoiding the opening, you could always look the other way and imagine that you were shaking hands with an embarrassed stranger—yourself.

Caring for my own children helped. My youngest son, now an adolescent, still enjoys a photo of me, dressed to the nines and holding him as an infant, with a patch of his vomit prominently displayed on the shoulder of my suit coat. He is amused by my lack of distress, then and now. And age (as well as my dogs) creates the same phenomenon that I experience in Chinese restaurants. Just as all the menu items seem to taste alike, so the body's various excretions and secretions—urine, feces, spit, sweat and the singular smell of childbirth—develop a common and less noxious valence with the passage of time. What once was foreign becomes familiar, and once familiar is a legitimate source for humor.

Pregnant mothers engage in their own imaginings. A private exchange, occurs between a mother and her unborn child. Few are privy to this silent process since it occurs in the closed spaces between mind and uterine darkness. Much is dreamed or intuited. Like the starling in Mary Poppins, who was fluent in the babble of pre-verbal twins, mothers, too, may conduct intra-uterine chats in the archaic tongues known only to them and their fetal companions. Conatact is delightful and quite the opposte of neurosis, as is much else in the world of gestation, much that might at first seem strange.

The loosening of mental processes seen in Cleo and Maureen rarely reaches such intensity and more rarely still crosses the line to madness. Still, many a pregnant mother feels estranged from her fetus, particularly during the first pregnancy. This sense of estrangement was captured in a charming manner during a research project I was involved in many years ago at the National Institute of Mental Health, where I spent two years involved in infant research. My friend and colleague Dr. Howard Moss and I interviewed fifty-plus primiparous mothers, both prior to and after birth. Their commonest dreams were filled with images of childbirth, but the delivery did not involve the naked, speechless, noisy, puzzling neonate. The dreamed infant emerged dressed like a toddler (shorts, shoes and all) who already walked, talked, and socialized. Yet with few exceptions, these new mothers adapted quickly to their roles as translators of their neonates' scrambled, wordless language.

In most pregnancies the resilience of the pelvic joints and the mental apparatus permit, with birth, a return to their original alignment. Little else remains but the slender stretch marks etched on memory and into the skin of an abdominal wall covering a now empty uterus. Life turns to more pressing matters: caring for a tiny, powerful, alien presence who has emigrated from familiar darkness to an unfamiliar shadow world, a presence that extends a mother's consuming passion from pregnancy into the light of day—a passion that D.W. Winnicott labeled "primary maternal preoccupation" that is no more nor less than falling in love.

A wise clinician once wrote that mourning and being in love are opposite sides of the same vital coinage, both sharing in common ruminations that crowd the mind, urgent longings to be with the one you love, be s/he newly arrived or newly departed. It is as if nature, in some quirky balancing act, some search for symmetry where there is none, matches the joy of our most precious gains to the sorrow of unbearable losses, and, in some kind of atavistic justice, lends proportion to the beginning and the end of days.

CHAPTER TWO: IN THE BEGINNING

For the error bred in the bone
Of each woman and each man
Craves what it cannot have,
Not universal love
But to be loved alone.

−W.H. Auden

Hal, a thirteen-year-old boy, was referred to me by his mother, who was concerned about his constant, increasing misery. He was perpetually griping: nothing was right, nothing fit, everyone mistreated him. He quickly alienated friends. "Unfair" was Hal's motto; his eyes were fixed upon the empty hole in the donut. Both mother and son appeared pale, underfed and rumpled. Hal's clothes were not quite clean and worn slightly askew. His blond hair was long, rarely cut and never combed. His blue eyes were somehow tired and lackluster. Mother seemed long-suffering and inwardly bitter, her petite, almost emaciated body a siren of silent but reproachful pain. In her interactions with her son she often appeared lifeless, glancing off his efforts to make contact. Hal's appealing features were usually suffused with a scowl, and he entered life, as well as my office, like nobility manqué, with an angry, arrogant litany of complaints: there was nothing to play with; the office was ugly and too hot, cold, or stuffy; I was boring, unable to understand his distress and wasting his time for the sake of his mother's money. His repeated question: "What can you do for me?" If life failed to change, and, of course, it could not do so to suit his terms, he would rather die, a fate he often and seriously considered in contemplating the empty shelves of his inner world.

A little of Hal went a long way with me. Children like him deplete one's stores. Despite all my good training, Hal tested my patience and altruism. I began to dread the times of our appointments, knowing that I could never satisfy his appetites, knowing that he would devalue my efforts, my usefulness, my adequacy. I became easily fed up with him. Had he been my own son, he would have felt my wrath long before this. At times my anger obscured the realization that he was showing me his world—a gaping mouth that turned every home-cooked meal into too little too late. From Hal, and many others in my work, I learned that there is more than one route to being special: one can be uniquely good or uniquely terrible, ugly, stupid—or under-served. Both poles are singular and serve a similar need to stand apart from all others, whatever the price (including death). The flip side of masochism is not sadism but narcissism.

In the beginning was not the word, only the speechless, raucous, self-centered self. Human character, to the extent there is one at the outset of life, shares its charm with more ugly sides. Infancy is dominated by greed, envy, voracious and immediate demands and murderous rage at frustration. All of these insatiable appetites rest precariously on the unswerving demand to be at the center of the universe, to be the only one. An infant's egocentrism is uncompromising. In the earliest months and years of life, not three but two is a crowd, and to the extent the outside world exists it does so to serve, promptly and precisely, the innate, inborn desire to be the one and only. More than many symptoms or syndromes, the gravitational pull of narcissism, insistent and resistant to change since it is both powerful and painless to its owner, serves as the underpinning of much unhappiness in childhood and later life. As a guide to one's future it is arrogant, impatient, rigid, omniscient, ignorant and unreliable. In a *New Yorker* cartoon an attractive couple is seated on a park bench, the man gazing at his reflection in an adjacent pond. His distraught partner asks, "Narcissus, is there someone else?" Narcissus, his youth and good looks not-withstanding, made big trouble for himself, ultimately drowning in his own reflected image as he indulged in its beauty. The lethality of this story line is in fact quite accurate. Gavin, an adult patient of mine, could only have sexual intercourse while looking at himself in the mirror. His intimate partner was himself, and while that was safe in one way, it left him totally alone. Despite several years of therapy, his growing sense of futility about change drove him ultimately to suicide. Suicide is one of the risks in this profession. I was aware of the depth of his despair, but there are times when the helper is helpless. His death continues to weigh on me—I wonder if there were ways by which I could have kept Gavin alive.

In most of us, the enduring demand to be the only one is grudgingly, reluctantly relinquished during the passage through childhood into adult life, in varying degrees traded in so that friendships, love and self-respect may play parts in our lives. In some, however, as can often be predicted by their childhood behavior, the habits of Narcissus persist, organizing the per-sonality more or less exclusively around self-interest, a sense of entitlement, rage, vulnerability to depression with suicidal and/or homicidal impulses and an inability to put one's self in another's shoes. Narcissistic children, Hal among them, act "special" but suffer frequent and often total collapse of their brittle self-esteem. They lack self-respect and experience an excess of shame, sensing their own fragility of self. Their iden-tity teeters uneasily, a rickety house of cards. The sturdiness and intactness of this shaky structure depend almost entirely upon validation of worth from the outside world: without ap-plause the show is a flop. Narcissistic children, like Hal, see themselves as treated unjustly by the world and tend to blame others for all of their misfortune, unable to see their part in determining the indignities they regularly suffer. One of my patients, an eighteen-year-old youth suffering his first episode of schizophrenia, put it poetically: "My eyes are turned inward." Many years later I understood that this was not an anatomical delusion but an accurate description of his consuming preoccupation with himself.

The narcissistic core wears many masks that may disguise its true colors: altruism, habitual self-denial, eating disorders, self-injurious behavior such as cutting, alcohol and/or drug abuse, and overtly psychotic phenomena reflecting a superabundance of narcissistic basalt, volcanic in origin, diamond-hard after cooling. Dana, a disarmingly mild and beautiful eight-year-old girl I saw in consultation, was plagued by morbid fears of what might befall her newborn and less than welcome brother, so much so that she hurried home after school, relinquishing friends and favorite activities, to stand guard at the door of her new sibling's nursery, protecting him from danger and lurking evil. Dana, unlike Gavin, was a sturdy youngster but, underneath all her outwardly altrusistic behavior, she struggled to remain sole proprietor of her parents' love.

Her apparent devotion, her new job description as security guard, was protecting her from her own envious fury. "Who," I asked, "would think of harming an innocent baby?" She shrugged. Encouraged, I tried a monologue: "Newborns are a pain; they keep you up at night and take up a mother's time. Most kids want to send them right back." She nodded vigorously, concurring. "It doesn't feel right to feel that way when everyone is oohing and aahing; it feels mean and nasty, but that's some of what all big sisters or brothers feel." Dana moved from my monologue to our dialogue. Thereafter, she and I determined that the evils were internal and the risks minimal. Anyone, we agreed, who says he or she wants to stop being the only one is fibbing big-time. She relieved herself of guard duty as she came to better accept the inevitability of murderous rivalry and her need to be the admired big sister, the one and only apple of her parents' eyes.

The origins of narcissistic difficulties in childhood are complex; they seem in part related to deprivation of sensible, empathic parenting, though as yet undocumented genetic and constitutional contributions must also exist. To mature with a healthy, necessary, and adaptive selfishness one needs to be parented with empathic hands that both give and take away, gratify and frustrate in the proper balance at the right times. Whether the infant-toddler's wishes and demands are granted immediately by parents who experience them as commands, are denied as if unreasonable, or are unheard, the end result can be a narcissistic child who feels entitled and/or unloved, unrecognized, uncertain of competence, dependent upon external affirmation while preoccupied with self to the exclusion of the surrounding world.

Spoiling is a well chosen, often prophetic metaphor. The child who suffers an excessive diet of indulgence and the unwarranted praise of psychological grade inflation, experiences, often permanently, wilting of the self's capacities for joy or contentment in a flawed world in which "...the imperfect is our paradise (Wallace Stevens)." Marla, a respected attorney, whom I saw for three years, with limited success, visualized a recurrent fantasy of a childhood birthday cake covered with green snot, her own. This brutal, accurate, nihilistic representation of her habitual need to devalue good times, good moods, good relationships and life accomplishments was a metaphor that fueled the more unhappy aspects of her life. "Who needs a baker like that?" I asked; "He would never pass muster with the Health Department and have a lot of sick, unhappy customers." She was not amused. Under the frosting, out of sight, was the working principle that "if I don't have everything, neither I nor anyone else will have anything." Buried even deeper lay the concern that, in an instant, "all I have can be lost." Marla and Hal took pages from the same book, though she, unlike Hal, never got beyond the Table of Contents.

Hal's pervasive sense of entitlement and grandiose expectations seemed to have their origins early in his life. His father, a charismatic alcoholic, abandoned the family shortly after his son's birth, leaving his already vulnerable mother clinically depressed and overwhelmed with the prospect of parenting alone and unloved. While devoted to Hal, she mothered him from afar, seeing him through a kind of haze. Having him as her only sustenance in life, she was loath to deny his wishes for fear he would turn on her. I had two victims for the price of one. I agreed to work with her son, meeting weekly with him and regularly with her. Taking on narcissism is hard labor; Hal was not an easy read for his mother, his peers or me.

At the outset of our therapy I experienced a brief honeymoon before Hal discovered that I was mortal. Coming in late for an appointment, I apologized to no avail: "Hal, I'm sorry, but I'm half an hour late; we can make it up next week." Silence, an angry glare and "You made me sit here. I've got better things to do than sit around waiting for this stupid meeting. I should have left, you should have called, you suck!" "Well," I said, "I hate waiting, too. It makes me feel like no one cares, and that's how you feel most of the time. But everybody needs room for things that come up, like for me today." Hal would have none of it: "You really do suck." Over the months of our weekly contact we experienced mounting frustration and despair, he with life, me with him. Hal's script in our sessions was repetitive, designed to fend off my patient suggestions by reducing them to rubble and me to helpless spectator of his demolition mode. My efforts to point out to him the connection between his insatiable wishes for everything and inevitable depression were met with scorn. My wondering if he missed having a father or a more responsive mother went unacknowledged. Helping him see that his need to "have it his way" put off friends, of whom there were few, fell upon deaf ears. To share, to consider the wishes of another was to lose his birthright. He seemed determined to retain his just due regardless of the cost. Coaching his mother in meeting his demands less agreeably was futile.

Freud opined that the sea was a symbol for mothers. Hal's one love was sailing and the ocean, about which he knew and taught me a good deal. At the time of his fourteenth birthday, having finally found a passion through which I might reach him, I wrapped and presented Hal with a small, beautiful replica of a sailing ship. It was opened hurriedly, without eye contact or enthusiasm, not acknowledged and abandoned or forgotten in a corner of my office as if it had never existed. My hurt and anger were hard to contain. When I remarked to Hal that my hurt feelings, which I shared with him, might mirror his own sense of being a devalued gift, a treasure thrown away, I was met with his usual derision.

Narcissism's vise-like grip is maddening to the therapist, fascinating as well, since its centrifugal determination to maintain itself flies in the face of logic, well-being and even life itself. A passage from J.M. Coetzee's annals of his own boyhood captures the essence of Hal's dilemma: "...he is still a baby...he tries to imagine his death...he tries to imagine the days wheeling around their course without him. But he cannot. Always there is something left behind, something small and black... dry, ashy, hard, incapable of growth but there. He can imagine himself dying but not disappearing...nothing can touch you, there is nothing you are not capable of. Those are the two things about him, two things that are really one thing, the thing that is right about him and the thing that is wrong about him at the same time. This thing that is two things means he will not die, no matter what; but does it not also mean he will not live? He is a baby...his mother holds him up before her [and] everything turns to stone and shatters...he is just a baby with a big belly and a lolling head, but he possesses this power." These are the maladaptive reaches of narcissism, its protective functions, its immutability, grandiosity, immortality, isolation and omnipotent, destructive fury. Clearly, so burdened, one cannot hope to live, love or find repose, forever dwelling in an Eden overrun with weeds. Yet for Hal, or any child burdened in this way, to leave this garden is to be stripped of one's only armor against a worse fate: to face an alien world stark naked—not indispensable but irrelevant, tiny and helpless, unimportant, unlovable, alone.

I have always loved geology. It studies the developmental history of earth. In my office are many rocks, crystals and fossils. Children are drawn to them. Road cuts of the earth's crust provide useful metaphors to students of childhood, with their lines of varying formations continuous, thick or thin, warped or straight, sometimes fractured and always of many, often beautiful colors. Such are the developmental lines of children as they move through life into adulthood. Continuity, interruptions, delays or, sometimes, arrest are evident. There is a time, somewhere between childhood and adult life, when the soft, malleable sediments of sandstone may metamorphose into impenetrable granite, when previously pliant traits may petrify into rigidities of character. I was concerned that Hal had reached that time and place.

His summer vacation interrupted sessions with me for some weeks. He spent this time in a beach home that he was fond of close to waters that he sailed. But as is sometimes the case in New England, this particular summer was unusually rainy, windy and cold, a risk well known and accepted by vacationers on Cape Cod and the Islands. Over those gray weeks Hal became increasingly depressed and intractably surly, at times telling his worried mother that he would welcome death's oblivion to escape his fate (the bad weather). In my office he greeted me with sullen reports of a sullied summer, both within and without: he expressed fury at the sun for not shining as he expected, a cosmic indignity that seemed central to his clinical depression and its nihilistic ruminations. Would any weather, any world, satisfy such an insatiable appetite I wondered out loud with Hal: "Where did you get the idea that the sun should shine for you? Not even the weathermen on Channel Seven can swing that one; wow, that's a humdinger!" His eyes met mine but he did not acknowledge my query. He took pencil and pad in hand, beginning to draw with intense concentration for some fifteen or twenty minutes.

The end product of his sketch was a ship, in fact a houseboat with one large room. The perimeter was lined with sumptuous goose-down pillows while the central space was configured as a gym with post and hoop at one end. At the other end of the room was a McDonald's snack bar that, Hal explained, was open twenty-four hours a day to serve the wishes of its sole customer. There were no human occupants, no one to interfere with his whims, no crew to navigate. Here was Hal's Twentieth Century version of the paradise he had lost. The sea was still, the sun eternally fixed at high noon in a cloudless sky. Here a boy need have no wants, no ungratified longings, none of the disappointments of life to cloud his view. Here was both cure and disease. He smiled when his work was completed. In some therapeutic efforts with children there are instances when, somehow, things come together, integrate or converge so that, however briefly, a window opens in a previously boarded up residence—a child trusts, approaches. This drawing brought me a visceral epiphany. The eagle had landed smack in the center of Hal's Garden of Eden.

I scanned his drawing intently and smiled in return. "This," I said quietly, "is what you want life to be, how the summer should have been." Hal's eyes filled with tears and he wept, convulsively, for some minutes, flooded with what seemed a great grief. In staccato fashion he offered for the first time his perception that his mother had never loved him, wished he had never been born, was a make-believe parent. He hated her empty gestures of affection; he hated her for what she was, and, more deeply, for what she was not. And he yearned for his father, idealized in his absence, who had stomached enough of both mother and son to disappear from view, an imagined rescue ship that saw neither shipwreck nor lifeboat before fading over the horizon. Through this catharsis Hal had moved from the generalities of his malaise to the specifics, however distorted, of his life. Just as a surgeon cannot treat abdominal pain without seeing the size, shape and condition of the belly's contents, I had needed Hal to openly acknowledge the realities of his life, past and present, to me and more importantly to himself. Now we could begin.

He had let go of something. His mother immediately sensed a greater openness and availability in her son and responded to it with more empathy than before. She felt valued and could, in turn, reciprocate. For the first time Hal was ready to ask and she could answer, replay and correct his missing father's narrative, reducing it to scale.

I sometimes let others do my work for me. I gave Hal a copy of an Isaac B. Singer short story, "A Fool's Paradise." In this wonderful parable a young man, about to marry, falls ill with a strange illness. No one can help until a Rabbi from afar, wise in the ways of the world, puts the young man to bed, dresses the servants as angels, and tells him he is dead and in Paradise where the wonderful menu is unchanging and his bed rest unrelieved. Soon he tires of this perfect, suffocating existence and returns to life, accepting if not embracing its imperfections and blessings. Hal read but offered no criticism on this tale. With me, however, he indicated that he was now better able to accept his mother's manner as the best she could manage. He saw that he could make her a better parent with his own behavior and that her deficiencies were hers rather than a response to his failings. He became more flexible with others and made a friend. His mood lightened. These modest shifts took many more months of work and did not excise the narcissistic core of Hal. But like the sea glass on Cape Cod, its sharp edges were rounded, less harsh, less likely to do harm.

Wise and experienced clinicians know that the capacity to be helpful to a child increases when one relinquishes the illusion of cure. I was helpful to Hal, though the ballast of his narcissism remained. Such modest successes are often all one can hope for. I am passionate about baseball and, as many of my patients know, often use its vicissitudes to bring perspective to children preoccupied with narcissistic perfection. I love to say that the very best hitters are out two thirds of the time and that in this game of life, the glorious grand slam is rare. Wee Willie Keeler, a tiny Hall of Famer, got there by "hittin 'em where they ain't." The inglorious bunt, well executed, sacrifices the batter for the team and brings the runner into scoring position, increasing his odds of coming home. In clinical efforts with children it is the bunt that matters. Up against narcissism there are no grand slams. And more often than not, one strikes out. I struck out with Larry.

Larry, some six years Hal's senior, lost his adoring mother at five years of age. This short, pudgy, intimidating, self-important young man was filled with dread. On an August Sunday in Hartford, his car stalled on Interstate 84 amidst back-to-back traffic. Standing on the center strip, cars streaming by, he suddenly felt totally alone, lost and convinced that no one could see him, no one would help him. He could barely contain the urge to leave this psychological Devil's Island by running into traffic and ending his torment, while at the same time dramatically punishing the negligent, uncaring passers-by, forcing them to witness his bloody demise. This was the ugly, drastic, dangerous work of Larry's narcissism and its trailer, the dread of abandonment. While his car was repairable, the faulty design of his psychological engine was not. Larry's entitlement was impenetrable, a barnacle-encrusted vessel hardened by the passage of years. The most we could manage was to make him more aware of his vulnerabilities, his extreme rejection-sensitivity, his blindness to others' needs, his own unreasonable neediness and the distorted rage that all of these might prompt in him.

To modify any aspects of narcissism in clinical work is a disappointing, Herculean task. Consider that Ebenezer Scrooge's therapists, the spirits of Christmas past, present and to come, were driven to show him Death itself, his own and Tiny Tim's, to gain his attention. It has always seemed to me that the brief sojourn of Adam and Eve in the Garden of Eden accurately parallels the amount of time each of us can legitimately spend, if we are reasonably lucky, in the normally egocentric phases of infancy and early childhood. Thereafter, the capacity to accept the vagaries of life on its own terms becomes an essential tool in coping with the sometimes bitter apples, the frustrations, disappointments and losses that are regularly and randomly handed out to us. The child who wants to remain in Paradise, or looks back upon it with longing, remains psychologically crippled: obsessed with being the one and only, mistaking heaven, so to speak, for the hell that it is. A wise colleague once commented that it takes children the longest time to want what they need: less, not more; something, but not everything. The grass, in Eden, is always browner.

Chapter Three: Of Human Bondage

Only Connect. – E.M. Forster

My days as an intern in pediatrics were long, my nights longer, and sleep either brief or absent. Especially after midnight the semi-darkness and silence pervading the usually frantic, well-lit hospital wards granted me temporary repose in an atmosphere of dim, fluorescent aloneness. Warmth at these times was welcome, reassuring. In the early morning hours of one such night, passing a crib on the toddler unit, I was assailed by the beseeching arms and Rossetti-like visage of a blonde, wide-eyed, two-year-old girl. Her insistent hugs seemed personal. But by the light of day she was a tiny, indiscriminate siren, promiscuously luring all who passed into her embrace, but soon moving on to the next comer with no deeper contact than a politician campaigning for office. Infection had brought her to the hospital, but her more serious, debilitating illness was a grave and permanent deficiency disease: the incapacity to attach to another, spawned in the early months of life by the psychological absence of her depressed and overwhelmed mother.

As with the Greylag Geese of Konrad Lorenz, there is a critical time period for human infants to connect to their caregivers. When this time passes without the process of attachment running its expectable course, impairments in trust, friendship and empathy result. Children suffering such "detachment" are everywhere and nowhere, unable to live well, love well, die well, or be alone. Relationships remain exploitive and need-fulfilling, serving an empty master whose internal attic contains few or no recorded images of being loved. As adults, these unfortunates fill their worlds with noise to quell the silence and emptiness within. They lack the capacity to be alone since they cannot soothe themselves with internal resources.

Karl, a superficially charming twenty-seven-year-old actor, an Alan Ladd look-alike, lived in constant dread of nights spent alone. He sought the physical company of any partner, male or female, who would sleep with him. These anonymous bed warmers were callously discarded the next morning after assuaging Karl's terror of aloneness for yet another night. After two or three sessions of psychotherapy, which he had sought in desperation at the time of his mother's death, he became aware that his hit-and- run mode of existence had been present since his earliest years. With my support (though it could have been anyone's) his acute pain diminished. At this point, however, he had no stomach for reflecting on the fleeting nature of his contacts as a problem; relief of immediate pain was enough. Since he remained fearful of genuine, enduring closeness, he jettisoned me, with predictable indifference, as another encumbrance to whatever he could garner in life. For Karl there were no connections. He was an adult version of the toddler whose crib I was unable to pass.

Since most children successfully form attachments during the first years of life, it is not the absence of connection but the rupture of these ties that composes the more common paradigm of loss, grief and mourning in childhood. The many symptoms and behaviors that children present, which are formally classified as illness, are often better understood and worked with by focusing on the centrality of loss or anticipated loss, for child, parent or both, rather than describing the more dramatic and less painful elements of the clinical profile. Separation and loss are signals; symptoms are noise. Grief sustained in childhood is remarkably intense when compared to its adult counterpart, both for the child and those around her. The child's tenuous defense mechanisms coupled with the unstable nature of the developing self account for the flood of emotion that loss or death in childhood unleashes. The thin lattices of being, like newly forming ice on a pond, come easily asunder. Denial of such pain in the observing adult is preferable to sinking into the frigid, salty waters of despair. It is no different with the elderly whom we often do not listen to, or if we do, whose painful, unedited truths we disregard.

When Beth's grief finally surfaced, I struggled to listen. Beth and her father adored each other. From birth through her first two years, their days began with the myriad rhymes, rituals and games loving parents invent and reinvent. A favorite involved her father wiggling her big toes while singing new ditties to his giggling, enraptured audience. Beth did not forget. On a business trip from Hartford to Washington, his car vaulted the guard rail. He died instantly. Like all two-year-olds, she had no cognitive tools, other than fantasy, with which to comprehend the incomprehensible or its aftermath. In childhood the death of a parent spawns two losses, the absent dead and the remaining but grief-stricken parent—another death, though in life. On the day of her father's death, and for many days thereafter, Beth's mother wept ceaselessly, overcome by her own pain, unable to respond to her daughter. Beth repeatedly mounted the living room couch, watching through the front window, waiting on her accustomed perch for her father's return. Increasingly puzzled and furious, Beth soiled the living room floor, a last straw to which her mother responded with understandable rage. Previously an impeccably clean youngster, Beth now soiled several times a day, bringing her to my care one year after her father's death.

At three Beth was a plucky, impudent gamin with long blonde

hair, finely chiseled features, and piercing green eyes whose gaze, quite independent of her prevailing mood, remained mischievous. While she wore an air of jaunty, self-assured insouciance, many years later she shared with me the terror and despair with which her inner, private world had been furnished. Still, she was acutely observant. In the waiting room, prior to my first visit with her, Beth spilled a bag of marbles she had in tow, a piece of home and comfort. Cleverly, I wisecracked that there was no better place to lose one's marbles. Twenty-five years later, she remembered. In transit to my office she took my hand easily. Like most tiny children, she looked downward, at her shoes or mine. She would also recall that view. Her chatter, head cocked, was full of the malapropisms of the young; it tinkled and charmed.

The child psychiatrist must recognize and respect boundaries. Children in need like Beth are especially vulnerable. She became very important to me and I to her. Devotion, concern and deep affection, in effect love, are indispensable elements for a psychotherapist. Neutrality, as described in the texts, is foreign to me. In my field the relationship is the central component of therapeutic success. However, a profession that deals in broken hearts requires its members to be alert to indulgence of their own needs, exploitation of those of their patients, or both.

Beth's fecal soiling was an anomalous symptom. The smell of feces or flatus is a universal icon of disgust. In childhood, anal matters are the basis of humor and embarrassment intense enough to deny one's own responsibilities for flatus and its smells. No normal child relishes being literally stinky or, derivatively, a stinker. But encopretic children, predominantly boys, seem oblivious to these powerful social conventions, willing to offend in any setting or circumstance without apparent awareness of the consequences; they are willing to sit in school, for example, with a mess in their pants until the teacher can no longer tolerate the smell. To further complicate matters, physical symptoms such as soiling that lodge in bodily sites, out of mind, are literally unspeakable. They cannot be translated into feelings or relationship problems; their somatic code cannot be broken, so they resist discussion in psychotherapy. Encopresis is notoriously insulated from language. Children will neither acknowledge nor converse about the obvious, the Emperor's new but soiled clothes.

Beth and I connected quickly. In the initial weeks of meeting with her there were no words or play that seemed related to her father. And while no direct information about her soiling surfaced, she focused attention on a Play-Doh factory that had the capacity to squeeze out long, messy cylinders of paste, a labor she industriously repeated until it became ritualized as the opening scene of every session. Beth also enjoyed finger painting, excitedly creating broad, thick swatches in black or brown but remaining stubbornly reluctant to identify the subject of her art when I was unwise enough to pursue its provenance. I assumed that these aspects of Beth's play related to her soiling and that she had been furious about her father's disappearance which her mother, wrapped in her own sorrow, had never explained. Did her now habitual messing signal an angry reproach toward her mother, who had not only taken her father away but neglected Beth since his disappearance? Did such profound distress on mother's part mean Beth had done something terribly bad, terribly wrong? I looked for answers to these questions in Beth's pictures, play and fantasies.

If these translations of her soiling were accurate, a straightforward, maternal apology was overdue. It was tendered, opening up a barrage of equally overdue questions on Beth's part: Where was daddy? Why didn't he come home? Wouldn't he come back if they called him? Didn't he like them anymore?

Or was he, like mother, angry that she had pooped on the floor, so angry that he was staying away to punish her? She knew that her mother had stepped into feces lying in her path and had seen the rageful result. For three-year-olds, chance and the uncertainty principle do not exist. Randomness is not credible: all events occur in a deterministic world within which the egocentric child is cause, the *deus ex machina*. As her mother and I answered these questions, Beth's soiling slowed, became intermittent and, after some weeks, stopped altogether, although tantrums seemed more frequent. In the office her fascination with Play-Doh and finger paint waned. But, cleaning up this aspect of her act did not bring her father home. Certainty that he would never willingly abandon her led to new hypotheses to account for his absence.

Classical Greek tragedies take their story lines from universal, developmental fantasies of childhood, beautiful for the clinician to witness, though often ghastly. Beth had seen her mother's rages repeatedly, at her father, at her. These crazed eruptions were terrifying. To Beth, mother was dangerous. Beth wondered if she was unbearably envious of a daughter's loving intimacy with father. No longer her husband's single love, had mother punished Beth, now a hated rival, by making certain that neither of them possessed him, magically destroying him? Such fantasized love triangles are the fabric of ancient myths such as that in which Clytemnestra murders Agamemnon, breaking Electra's heart. Much great art, of whatever medium, emerges from the creator's transformation of such real life dramas as separation, reunion, rivalry and loss. To Beth this patricidal script was real. Sadly, when fantasies and external reality mirror one another, the imagined takes on the quality of fact. Closeness to men became hazardous to Beth, proximate to lurking disaster and death. She played out these concerns with dollhouse figures in my office for some months. But such efforts were not sufficient to protect her from her past, her future or her imagination.

I worked with Beth for two years. What I assumed was the final phase of our therapy dealt with the persisting enigma of mortality. The understanding that death is permanent is rarely accomplished before the age of nine or ten. Beth, at age five, had neither attended her father's funeral nor visited his grave. She struggled to digest her father's death without success. It seemed that Easter, the season of death and transfiguration, would never come in her fourth year; winter was bitterly persistent. In the midst of preparing the eggs for the family hunt, Beth told her mother that she wanted her father to be in attendance. She dictated an invitation, asking her mother to share it with me:

Dear Dr. Robson,

I want to say that I love him. I want to say that I'm going to send an Easter card to him. Now I want to tell him that we're going to send another Easter card to him from my mommy. We're going to Washington and we'll see him in the spring. Can't go now because it's too cold and windy.

Love,
Beth

Her signature was spread in bold letters across the page, the "h" lying, somewhat forlornly, on its side.

Some weeks later, without warning, in the midst of a session with me, Beth interrupted her play, stood transfixed, eyeing me from across the room, and uttered in a barely audible voice: "My daddy is in a box in the ground. He can't eat, he can't talk and he doesn't wake up." I nodded silently, flooded with her sadness and my own tears. I reminded Beth that neither

her soiling nor love for her father had led to this unhappy, still partially grasped reality.

Soon thereafter I stopped seeing Beth and her mother. It was a natural time for interruption, as the fog surrounding her loss was lifting. Four years later (she was now nine), I met Beth again. By chance she, her mother and I were attending the same holiday party. I was delighted to see them and to learn that Beth was apparently doing well. Her mother turned to Beth and asked, "Do you remember Dr. Robson?" Beth shyly turned to me and nodded no. Then, peering down at my shoes, her prevailing view of me at three, she surveyed me again from my soles to my head, nodded in the affirmative, and smiled. Shoes made the man.

Losses such as Beth sustained distort relationships and reality. Parting in certain situations can even be lethal. This is particularly true for the victims of asthma, "the illness of terror." For the afflicted child a serious attack simulates suffocation, or drowning. For the parent of such a child, the random onset and danger of attacks creates an attachment demanding more or less constant apprehension and scrutiny. Separation is one of several situational stressors that can precipitate symptoms, leaving parent and child perpetually in fear of parting. Psychotherapy in these circumstances revolves around strengthening the sense of mastery and competence in the child. Tod was a severe asthmatic. Afflicted since age four, he was ten when I was asked by his pediatrician to reduce his mother's anxiety. Medical control of his attacks was poor; he had entered the hospital on multiple occasions with his breathing seriously compromised. His parents had struggled to maintain a sense of normalcy in Tod's life and their own. I was struck by Tod's own efforts in that direction: he appeared a robust boy with a warm smile. He dressed like his peers. He loved Elvis.

But his moon face, a product of chronic use of corticosteroids, and barrel chest, resulting from increasing efforts to maintain normal breathing, gave notice of his illness. The goals of therapeutic efforts with Tod and his family were aimed at his gradually assuming more responsibility for anticipating attacks and administering medication before his wheezing reached dangerous levels. At night, in darkness and separated from his mother, he felt especially vulnerable. By morning he often ended up at the foot of his parents' bed in the sleeping bag kept there as an outpost of safety. While slow progress was evident, the acceleration of his disease led to a decision on his pediatrician's part to send Tod to a hospital in Arizona. There he was to remain, separated from his parents, for months or longer. Anticipating the dread of this decision, I saw both Tod and his parents more often as the departure date approached. He was to travel to Tucson with a nurse but no family members. He managed a wan smile the day prior to his departure. I was called that evening by the Emergency Room near Tod's home. Tod had arrived there *in status asthmaticus*—a state of uninterrupted asthmatic attacks. Tod was carried into the hospital and died several hours later. "Parting," Emily Dickinson wrote, "is all we know of heaven and all we need of Hell." Tod's funeral, which I attended, seemed dream-like and muted, cast in the pastels of a Fellini film. I shared in the family's sorrow.

His parents, with whom I had established a close relationship, asked to meet with me shortly after his death. Grieving, guilty and angry, they wondered what they or anyone involved in Tod's care could have or should have done. Already they were discussing having another child, a course of action I strongly discouraged, knowing that children who replace a dead sibling fare poorly in many instances, both they and their parents haunted by the ghost of an unknown, larger-than-life, idealized presence with whom they cannot complete and are sometimes confused. Some five years later Tod's parents sought me out again. They had a new son, now four, who was born, almost to the day, on the second anniversary of Tod's death. He had just developed early symptoms of asthma. Driven by the unbearable loss of their son, this second chapter of a sad book reconfirmed my professional impotence in the face of a fated or ill-fated drama. This visit from his parents also highlighted an unfortunate pattern of human behavior: the powerful tendency to repeat or reinvent past traumas. Freud called this "the repetition compulsion."

Beth's life went forward. Her mother remarried a decent man who reached out to his new step-daughter. But, convinced of the dangers of that closeness by her father's death, she resisted her own longings, staying at arm's length from him as she entered puberty and adolescence. The bad cards of fortune are not always random: her step-father died from acute leukemia. Later I met Beth, now twenty, in a hospital parking lot. She was pregnant and married. Our contact was fleeting. Then, at the age of thirty she asked to meet with me. Now a tall, slender woman dressed in black, her eyes were instantly recognizable, as if the three-year-old I'd known so well lingered, unchanged by time, living within an adult's body like the smallest figure in a Russian doll. Her seeking me out was a kind of homecoming for both of us. She was in deep distress, desperate and suicidal. A well-meaning therapist, after hearing her life story, had insisted that she visit, for the first time, her father's grave to "begin healing." This misguided effort unleashed a torrent of memories and dreams in Beth: bodies rising from the earth as in *Revelations,* unresolved feelings and memories flooding her days and nights. Mistrust of closeness to men continued to plague her despite her husband's apparent reliability. She had borne two children but they, it seemed, mothered her. My thrill at seeing Beth after so many years was tempered by the depth of the psychological scars she bore, and by my recognition that my work with her had not diminished the power of more malignant strains in her life. A favorite nostrum of one of my old teachers, an auto mechanic before he entered medical school, was "We don't make 'em, we just service 'em." A candid reminder of my profession's limitations.

I was able to facilitate Beth's resumption of therapy and support her accepting the care she sought but feared. Her life had been difficult. Her many wounds remained open and raw. She took the presence of her pain as a reminder that she should look backwards, exhume her father and her memories of her earliest years. This mission had already proven hazardous to Beth, and I warned her that it might be safer and more helpful to quiet the troubled waters of her present life before seeking to calm the stormy seas of her past. Some days after Beth's visit I received a package: a bag of marbles and a note that read: "I haven't lost them yet." Beth lives in me just as I live in her. Her marbles and her note, now framed, sit on my office desk, a precious connection linking present to past with timeless, bittersweet memories and a shared sorrow in both our hearts.

If one views the practice of child and adolescent psychiatry as a musical composition, it would read "theme and variations." The central needs of human life are few: to be healthy, to be loved, to be competent at some form of endeavor, to be able to laugh and to play. The variations on these themes comprise the beauty of the field, each presentation the same but different, the differences highlighting the elegant nuances and overtones that ultimately draw one back to the center. Monet painted one haystack many times and Cezanne one Mt. Sainte-Victoire. In my field, attachment, separation and loss are played as the opening bars by the French horn and are repeated by the strings in a coda's closing notes.

Chapter Four:
Male and Female Created He Them

The Phoenix riddle hath more wit
By us; we two being one, are it;
So, to one neutral thing both sexes fit.

– John Donne

Mason was somebody's darling. That was clear the moment I saw him. Here stood a well-scrubbed, verbally precocious three-year-old with carefully groomed, blond hair. He strutted briskly and pompously about while scanning his surroundings with a penetrating, skeptical gaze. Dressed in expensive, slightly mannered but tasteful outfits, he pranced and gestured with the flourishes of a French courtier. Daily, at his preschool, he separated from his anguished mother with melodrama straight from *The Perils of Pauline*, twisting and turning in her arms, while in protest he was dragged to the school door. Once amputated and safely ensconced in his schoolroom, Mason moved to the dress-up corner where, for the remainder of the morning, he donned skirts, hats, scarves, jewelry and any other available accoutrements of female fashion. What served as entertainment for his peers was a vocation for Mason. The daily reenactment of this tragi-comic scene led Mason's pediatrician to suggest to mother that she seek consultation.

He approached my office with surprising assurance, summarily dismissing his astonished mother at the door. Cocking his head like a miniature late night talk show host or master of ceremonies, Mason perused me carefully and opened with: "So you are my unusual friend." Introductions completed, he gravitated to and carefully explored the dolls on my shelves, ignoring trucks, guns and building blocks. He told me of his collection of some forty Barbie dolls, gifts from a doting grandmother who could never say no. I was eager in this initial meeting to begin exploration of Mason's gender preference by seeking out masculine ambitions that might be concealed, for safety's sake, beneath the surface of his feminine persona. Certain developmental anxieties in boys often lead to withdrawal from or disguising of male identity, a flight from "manliness" driven by a sense of danger. In such cases the clinician's task is to reduce the child's dread while freeing up authentic strivings. But if the gender preference seems fixed and fundamental to a child's core identity, the task is clearly different and involves helping child and parents live with the atypical while navigating the shoals of a predictably intolerant world.

Mason turned to the future, sharing his visions of adult life. His father was president of a successful company. Like father, unlike son? Mason dreamed, uneasily, sharing "and when I grow up I want to be a pr... pr... pr...princess." His *pr's* suggested the notion that president was at least present in a rudimentary fashion, and his stuttering and stumbling over this word revealed his anxiety. But as time passed, it became clear that Mason, free in my space to be and become whomever he wished, was unambiguously committed to life as female royalty, a princess and not a president.

The developmental line of gender and sexuality is marked by four nodal points along its sometimes treacherous traverse from birth to adolescence—biological gender; core gender identity (the inner, subjective perception of being male or female, the contours of which are definitively shaped by three years of age); sex role (the culture's stereotypical patterns and characteristics of boy/girl, man/woman behavior); and, finally, sexual orientation (preference for a male or female sexual partner). For the most part these points are congruent with one another over time, though many permutations appear as they do in all of nature's enterprises. The internal crystallization of core gender identity is not determined by biological gender alone. Rather, it emerges from a complex interplay of genetic, constitutional, familial and cultural influences. Most gay men have male core gender identities. Boys like Mason, biologically male, psychologically female, may live out their lives suffering intensely, never feeling like themselves or who or what they want to be. There is a complete, restless, impatient homunculus living within, a cross-sex homunculus driven into hiding by societal forces, externally conforming to the culture's sex roles but longing to emerge. In the normal course of development through the early years, both children and their parents can struggle mightily with these complex and emotion-laden issues, more harshly and rigidly perhaps in this culture than some others. Males, the most vulnerable sex both biologically and psychologically, may struggle harder. It is interesting that embryologically the female genitalia is basic to all fetuses, the male machinery a later add-on and psychologically less securely fastened. Tomboy girls are tolerated if not venerated in contrast to effeminate boys, who are relentlessly persecuted by their anxious, threatened peers. One such patient of mine recalled being tied to a tree by neighborhood boys and made to cry out for his mother when seven or eight years of age. This childhood rendition of "gay-bashing" seems mild compared to the murderous rage of adolescents and young adults who are burdened by unresolved gender issues. During my training in Boston, male teens for Saturday night entertainment sought out gays in their gathering places, frequently breaking jaws or limbs in their frenzy to disown any female characteristics of their own. Happily, American culture has become more tolerant of gender ambiguity and has blurred, to some extent, the line between the sexes. When normally aligned, the gender components of the developing self in children are relatively silent; but their influence upon the course and well-being of a life are starkly evident when their natural order is disrupted.

Jacob, a fifteen-year-old, was raised in an Orthodox, Jewish home. From age seven or so, he suffered from chronic depression, which became so profound as he entered puberty that he required inpatient hospitalization, the setting where I first met him. A gangly boy with a shock of unruly dark hair, he shuffled and usually averted his gaze in social encounters. He had become persistently suicidal, feeling that life had become overwhelmingly bleak. The intense religiosity of his family lent him little comfort, adding harsh, intolerant judgments to his sense of unworthiness. While early-onset depression is not rare in children, the causes are usually discoverable. With Jacob I remained puzzled, feeling that the gravity of his depression did not fit with other aspects of his life. He responded poorly to psychotherapy and anti-depressant medication. Sessions with him seemed unproductive. After eighteen months with little progress evident, Jacob looked me in the eye and haltingly confessed: "I want to be a woman." His encounter with an age mate who wore earrings and lipstick to school had prompted the timing of this revelation.

A new set of problems now emerged as the ripples of his disclosure spread. Strife, humiliation and shame within his family and his school surrounded and closed in on Jacob, who had quickly learned that truth has consequences and that the social contract was not written for him. The solution he had longed for brought him new misery rather than emancipation, isolation rather than community. To fully embrace the transsexual world, he wanted sex-change surgery but knew that five or so years would have to pass before he was old enough for that option. His depression and suicidal despair continued. The suicide rate in boys like Jacob is significantly higher than the already elevated incidence during adolescence. Dressing, when permitted, like a woman and now called Janice, Jacob could neither retreat to his former self nor advance to his new identity and its sub-culture. Helplessness to change one's fate is depression's bedfellow. I lent Jacob support but that was too little. The discomforts of his daily life validated his despair.

I was hopeful that intervening at such an early age with Mason might spare him the vicissitudes of Jacob's adolescence. My cautious optimism failed to fully recognize the profound antipathy with which society approaches any deviations in sex or gender in its members. In the office Mason initially tested my tolerance for his preferences: wrapping his head in turbans or affecting a woman's voice, he scanned my face for signs of disapproval. Shortly, he felt sufficiently safe to bring his feminine longings regularly to me. And once aware that his identity was female, his parents lent their support at home. But out in the world his increasingly open desires to move, dress, talk and play like a girl complicated his school life and friendships, leading to a sequence of increasingly complicated decisions.

How, for example, does one guide a child and his parents when at five a boy insists on wearing feminine attire into a gender-specific world? I knew that Mason faced many years of living in a stereotypical male society, perhaps a decade or more, before any version of coming out would be acceptable. Should he be encouraged to fashion a male sex role so as to get along in the world, or would that direction crush the self that was genuine? Should I recommend a single sex or co-ed school for him, given that there were no environments tailored to trans-sexual children? I opted for a traditional, all-male school whose administration seemed sensitive to Mason's plight. Mason was now six and our paths diverged. I moved to Washington, DC to join the Public Health Service for two years. I referred my unusual friend to a colleague for ongoing care. However, his future and mine would cross again.

As a child psychiatrist I was often consulted by the Court or agencies with questions as to the fate of children raised by gay or lesbian parents. The irrational national controversy over this family structure generated great heat based on no light. In fact, all existing studies of such children find no increase in gay or lesbian life preferences when compared to the offspring of traditional male-female parents, not a surprise since the vast majority of gays and lesbians develop within "straight" families. The issue of sexual orientation in parents arose in my treatment of Emma. Unlike Mason, Emma was a spunky, delightful seven-year-old when I first encountered her. Cute but feisty, she shook her decidedly feminine pigtails when irked, a not uncommon mood. While her gender identity seemed secure, her world was not. One of three children, she shared her time between her parents whose relentless conflict dominated Emma's world.

Her father, unbeknownst to her, conducted a secret life as a transsexual. When Emma was three, he returned home one evening dressed in heels, stockings, a dress, rouge, lipstick and a wig. Stunned by this metamorphosis, Emma, who was not forewarned, exhibited confusion and anxiety, initially solving her dilemma by assuming that her father was playing a practical joke, a kind of out-of-season Halloween prank. But her father, hoping to become the best and only parent in his daughter's life, told her "Your daddy is dead; you have two mommies now." This self-serving revelation stunned her mother, too, and led to Emma's referral to me in the turmoil that followed. In my office she played out with hand puppets and tiny family figurines the black comedy of her family drama. Time and again, in fury, she threw the father figure across the room, often exclaiming that this "mommy-daddy" was bad and mean. Of course, she loved her father, felt rejected and abandoned by him, sensing the tectonic plates of her life shifting precipitously. Her mother, a kind and competent parent, feared the worst for Emma if she was parented by this strange and unnatural apparition who was her father. She sued for divorce and requested a custody study that recommended sole residence with her. As Emma's world reformed, it was evident that her feminine identity had robustly withstood any and all assaults upon it.

By the age of nine she was managing well and had pushed out of conscious awareness most recollections of those traumatic years. Memory, the trickster, is on occasion kind. Her mother remarried, and Emma moved to a new state hundreds of miles away, where she thrived. Her mother wrote me when Emma was eighteen. She was in college and a gifted short story writer. Emma never spoke of her father and seemed to have no memories of him.

In some circumstances, children with firm core gender identity appear to vest themselves in the ways of the opposite sex. This is the rule with tomboys but not with their male counterparts. It was, however, true of Harold. A strapping ten-year-old with Tom Sawyerish freckles and red hair, Harold sat in my office and assertively corrected me, after I greeted him by his given name: "Call me Margaret." In child psychiatry the work sometimes presents one with Rosetta Stones that require efforts to break the code. I will often have children introduce me to their worlds by drawing their homes. Harold readily did so, leaving one room unfurnished, untouched. I asked about this design omission and he slowly, haltingly told me that this was his sister Margaret's room. She had died of cancer several years before and Harold, the sole surviving child, had witnessed and was immersed in his mother's descent into hell that this tragic, untimely death precipitated.

Margaret's room, with all of her personal belongings untouched, was sealed and in effect became her mausoleum. No one in the family spoke of her. But Harold, in an effort to bring his mother back to him, found what seemed to him the simplest solution by taking on his dead sibling's name. The failure of his mission, and the concern it raised in those who loved him, led to a more enduring refurnishing of the family home, both internally and externally; and as Margaret's passing was more appropriately mourned, the shades in her bedroom were raised and Harold was free to reclaim his name, his gender and his life.

Mason's mother called me when her son was thirteen. She reported that Mason sought the company of gay youth and appeared at home in that world. But his course through childhood was stormy and friendless. Ten years later, while writing this book, I asked Mason, now Marissa, to meet with me. Tall and "twiggy thin," she was dressed in jeans rather than traditional female attire. Her henna-tinted hair framed but was incongruous with the eyes, smile and tone of voice of Mason at six. Marissa resembled a man in drag more than a woman. While eager to meet with me and tell her story, Marissa was wary and good contact was difficult to establish, as had been the case many years earlier. She lacked animation; the histrionic liveliness of earlier years was absent. She seemed mildly depressed or empty. I learned that Marissa had undergone castration four months prior to our meeting and was now on female hormones, the final phase of her conversion.

The prospect of meeting Mason had been exhilarating to me. I suppose my patients carve out a space somewhere within that remains furnished but unoccupied in their absence. But this meeting with Mason left me depressed. I was humbled and saddened by the lackluster outcome of his/her tarnished life. I sensed that little ordinary pleasure would ensue. I wished I could have done more. His school-age years had been painful. At twelve, homoerotic feelings had surfaced, leading to a series of casual relationships with gay men. In the years that followed, Marissa continued to have relationships with men, most of them short-lived. She feels her own gender status is now settled, though her personal identity remains a work in progress. Marissa's mother feels that her son is desperately lonely, moving from one emotional crisis to another. What struck me most about my meeting with Marissa was the emotional distance at which it was conducted: I suffered through a joyless and impersonal interview with a gender-amorphic and unformed stranger well known to me in her childhood. Her fantasies of femininity at three may have brought her more joy than life as a woman with all its complexities. Without the ongoing support of her devoted parents, it is hard to see how she could manage her shadowy life.

The social contract is exacting, entering the awareness of children very early in life. They know that a fundamental stipulation of this contract involves conformity with one's biological gender. The author of *Genesis* made such conformity seem far simpler than it is; we are not just created man and woman. The long path to self-certainty, the unchanging sense of "I," cannot be accomplished without gender certainty, and that path is frequently steep and sometimes impassable.

CHAPTER FIVE: UNHOLY LOVE

Her parthenogenetic birth from Adam's body makes Eve his daughter so that the Judeo-Christian tradition rests on a primal father-daughter incest motif. – Naomi Goodman

Tess loathed her husband's body: his long muscular torso, hirsute back, and, especially, his genitals. A hug or caress from him set her on edge, filled her with apprehension and disgust at the prospect of sexual intimacies. In her fifth year of marriage, she was the mother of three young children. After the birth of her first child, intercourse became painful then repugnant. Over time she began to avoid all physical contact with her husband who, though a gentle, somewhat passive man, was increasingly puzzled and hurt. A tall, buxom woman, Tess was flirtatious, quietly seductive in her public persona. She longed for extra-marital affairs, "sex without complications." Privately, she showed occasional flashes of self-deprecating humor but more often was grimly intense. While referred initially for her chronic depression, she soon revealed how fully her attitudes toward sex with her spouse preoccupied her, leading to serious reflection on divorce. To abhor sex with him was, increasingly, to abhor the totality of his presence in her life.

As Tess explored with me the history of her sexuality, the dynamics of her family of origin became more transparent. Her mother was a brittle, self-centered woman with limited capacity for warmth, while the father, handsome and ebullient, was open and spontaneous with his loving, possessive feelings for his daughter. It was he who had provided the swaddling embraces that Tess craved. At twelve Tess was lectured by her father on the dangers of dating, of naive trust in what was the sexually exploitive intent of most males. Standing sternly over her, crowding her, he began to fondle her buttocks. She was frozen, stunned. The details of this scene were scorched into her memory: her father's sweaty smell, his breathing, his flushed ruddy face, the feel of his hands on her flesh, the heat of it all. His fondling continued through Tess's early adolescent years. Her only means of preserving the closeness to him now was to paint over this inexplicable violation with psychological whiteout, eliminate it from conscious awareness. Like most abscesses, it remained encapsulated until her marital sex life began. Then, fragment by fragment, it drained, surfaced and reassembled itself in consciousness. Her now unedited memory, like a pornographic film strip, became the focus of her attention during foreplay and penetration with her husband, fusing so that memory and partner, father and husband, past and present became one, filling Tess with repulsion and dread. So powerful was this perception that during their infrequent sexual encounters, Tess began to silently repeat to herself a mantra: "You're not my father, you're not my father."

In therapy we struggled to make sense of her father's startling behavior. Tess's rage flowered and spread, like poison gas, to all men except her sons, whom she idealized and physically "loved to death." Try as I might to separate her past paternal relationship from her marriage, boundaries would not rise. The time warp of memory had petrified. She tired of such painstaking work. Her depression deepened, she seriously considered suicide but opted for a grave but less lethal option: initiating divorce proceedings. She abruptly withdrew from her therapy against my advice. Her husband had become the repository of all that was bad and, leaving him, she again preserved her present relationship with her supportive father whom she chose not to confront with his prior behavior. Tess moved to the deep South, taking with her the burden of her frightened, twelve-year-old self, very much alive within, but not well. She remarried, though I do not know the course of her new life. I do know that Freud was correct in asserting that character is destiny and that Tess's future remained bound to her past.

The erotic and sexual aspects of children's lives are obscured in the shadows of society's anxiety and denial; incestuous relations are especially alarming. From Freud to Sophocles, such impulses have been seen as the stuff of high drama and psychic torment but rarely as natural, necessary, useful partners to self and gender-development. While sexuality is central in human affairs, there is a tendency to view the erotic life of children prior to puberty as either absent or as harmless play, and puberty as a biological stranger, a sudden, ill-fitting visitation without past or future, arriving uninvited from parts unknown. The idea that there is a complex, continuous evolution to the sexual life of children, beginning with birth itself, is seen as an aberrant belief of cranks and perverts. But if comfort with one's physical self, sensuality, sexual arousal and safe, modulated, loving closeness are not learned as unified parts of a whole in infancy and childhood, they invariably remain isolated from one another thereafter. Such is the reason that in adult life the comfortable union of intimate relatedness and sexuality is all too often not accomplished. These are two crucial competencies more often evolving as independent, unrelated, parallel developmental trajectories that go their separate ways. The psychological chasm between intimacy and sexuality, evident in Tess, is present in myriad failed relationships and contributes significantly to human loneliness, estrangement and difficulty sustaining long-term connections with a partner.

The child psychiatrist, if he or she can tolerate what is clearly in view, is witness to this developmental line of sexuality as it unfurls within the child and his family. Like other developmental phenomena, emerging sexuality is determined by genetic influences, temperament, parent-infant interaction and social mores. At one end of that curve lie emotional constriction and inhibition of eroticism; at the other extreme, one finds incest and/or sexual abuse. These polar opposites both lead to developmental impairments. Between these extremes, over a long continuum, one finds both the many varieties of healthy sexuality and the common but highly malignant sexual over-stimulation of children, perhaps less visible but more damaging to the developing child's capacities than incest or abuse. No engine, no developing ego, can run when persistently flooded. The common sources of such unmodulated, sensory overload include constitutional inability to "gate out" or filter incoming stimuli and/or family lifestyles that are intense, arousing and uninsulated. Such stimuli and lifestyles produce children who are like pianos without damping pedals. Parental empathy and accommodation to an infant's particular style and temperament are essential in fostering self-regulation and control, porcelain-coating the overheated wires of developing sexuality.

As noted above (see Chapter One) what Winnicott called "primary maternal [parental] preoccupation" with newborns is in fact being in love. He saw this state as essential for both parent and infant attachment and later life outcomes. He did not discuss the inseparable connection between the arousal of wishing to fuse and merge with the other and the sexual desire that is part of being in love at any age. The nuzzling, caressing, cuddling, cooing, biting, stroking and sucking between mothers and their infants reappear as the foreplay of adult sexual relatedness. A small sub-group of normal mothers come to orgasm when nursing. Only in our species is the breast both a source of nourishment and an organ of sexual arousal. If incestuous impulses were not powerful, the rigid societal taboos against them would not exist. I have wondered whether their presence, when appropriately governed, can be considered adaptive in our species, facilitating both durable attachment of parents to their young as well as successful melding of intimacy and sexuality in the developing infant and child. Incestuous desires become maladaptive at either end of the bell-shaped curve: when anxious, constricted adults recoil from physical contact with their young or, conversely, have or exercise insufficient control over those same impulses, as with Tess's father. The curriculum for the coming together of intimacy and sexuality begins at birth. Its healthy completion depends upon the psychological integrity, capacity for restraint and respect for boundaries with which parents raise their young.

Winnicott also described two distinct modes of contact between parents and their offspring: the "orgiastic" style characterized by over-stimulation, lack of interpersonal boundaries and overwhelming excitement, in contrast to the empathic, balanced, low-intensity, and respectful "object-relatedness." A bell-shaped curve connecting these modes describes the spectrum of human parenting styles. I grew up in Illinois, a farm state where children of twelve or thirteen had to drive tractors. Recognizing the hazards of puberty and speed, it was customary to affix a wooden block appropriately called a "governor" under the gas pedal. All children, and many parents, need governors. Tess's father lacked one; Ben needed one.

Ben, the oldest of three children, was five when referred by a terrified pre-school director. This robust, handsome, reckless, ebullient boy ravaged the girls in his group by regularly grabbing them in the crotch. Angry, anxious parents let it be known that Ben was on the do-not-invite list and threatened to remove their children unless immediate action was taken. That action brought Ben to my attention. In my office he lost little time in demonstrating the problem. He was a whirling dervish whose actions spoke louder than words. He lay supine on the floor, mimicking copulatory thrusts. His drawings rendered crude figures with disproportionately large breasts and penises, and he related to me with intense, boundary-violating physicality. His parents were bright and devoted to Ben, and while consciously eager to calm his alarming firestorm they were at a loss to explain it. My questions regarding bathing and toileting practices, privacy, modesty and the physical stimulation involved in greetings and partings met with blank looks. Both parents assured me that Ben was not excited at home, a sign of their denial or the common disorder of parental blindness. Considering ADHD (Attention-deficit Hyperactivity Disorder) an aspect of his difficulty, I started him on Ritalin. His teachers reported some motor-slowing, but his wandering hands continued to be a problem.

In our sessions I involved Ben in quiet games, attempting to cool his ardor. But he was already addicted to action. With miniature family figures he played out repeated scenes of lust, violence and frenzy that reflected the unquiet nature of his inner world. The images he drew continued to exhibit sexual themes. After some months of what felt to me like fruitless effort, I was becoming discouraged. Then, as if it was an entirely new notion, Ben's mother, musing with me in the office, wondered whether her nuzzling and kissing him passionately on the stomach, a nightly bedtime ritual, bothered Ben at all. The belatedness of her revelation was not conscious withholding of important information. Rather, her bedtime ritual had become habit, caused no pain, and was deeply gratifying to mother and son. Further, to give it up would establish greater distance from Ben and foster his separation from her. With stakes this high, this painful, it is often the case that such observations as Ben's mother made never reach a point of open discussion, never come to light. But if they do, a new phase of treatment is often heralded. In Ben's case his parents were beginning to see that their over-stimulating behavior related to Ben's sexualizing activities. They worried, appropriately, about

Ben's siblings and became more vigilant about the interactions of the children with one another.

The stalled therapeutic process began to move. Ben's father took notice of his wife's morning exercises conducted daily on the living room floor, in her nightgown, breasts and genitals exposed to Ben's excited, exploring gaze. She, in turn, caught sight of Ben's fascination with his father's penis which was visible when his skimpy, after-bath towel covered little of its intended target. Once these rituals, long out of parental awareness, were illuminated, other similar, sexually arousing practices poured forth into the light of day where they became subject to modulation. The orgiastic was moving toward ego-relatedness. These sexually provocative behaviors illustrate the extraordinary extent to which eroticism is imbedded in normal, everyday parenting. Ben quieted, his self-control began to organize and restrain the impulses that had flooded him; his mastery rewarded him, the praise of his teachers adding support to his progress. At age eighteen Ben was a gifted student who imagined a career as a trial lawyer. He was accepted for early admission to a prestigious college. The runaway energies of his early years had been harnessed.

There are those occasions when a brief therapeutic foray is sufficient to reset a family's thermostat of stimulation. Diana, a nine-year-old girl with blonde braids and pale skin, was the daughter of an accountant who himself had grown up in a physically constricted, oppressive home where physical contact was discouraged. Determined to spare his children this legacy, he shed his clothes. Nightly on returning home from work, he calmly conducted his family's life in the nude. I learned of this paternal practice from Diana who was referred to me because of her extreme anxiety, her hand-wringing worry. In her picture of the family home she drew a scene at first unintelligible: a second floor room with what turned out to be a hole in the floor though which she and her brother listened to and watched parental intercourse on enough occasions to impress them. The sight of parental love-making and the sounds of orgasm are terrifying to children who confuse the scene and acoustics of passion with murder. A good carpenter and discussion of the values of paternal modesty reduced Diana's intolerable levels of arousal. The record for speedy interventions of this kind was set by a seasoned, Viennese teacher of mine. His anxious, agitated, eight-year-old patient achieved repose when the intercom between the parental bedroom and their child's was turned off at night, thereby eliminating alarming sounds and anxiety.

The reversible damage of overstimulation contrasts with the developmental malformations resulting from serious abuse. Martha, referred in the context of a criminal case against her stepfather, was also nine. But, unlike Diana, this slightly overweight girl with thick glasses was almost mute. She related with difficulty, turning and glancing away from me, speaking rarely and in a barely audible voice. Having lived with her mother and stepfather for the last two or three months, she had recently told her disbelieving mother of her stepfather's regular sexual approaches to her during her mother's absences from home, shopping or bowling with friends. The stepfather was immediately removed from the home, pending a full investigation of which my evaluation was a part.

In a dull monotone, Martha blandly described lurid details of his quiet but intimidating insistence that she undress, spread her legs and let him play "Push" with her, inserting his erect penis into her vagina. Afterwards he cleaned his semen from her genital area in the adjacent bathroom with towels whose colors and patterns Martha could describe in detail. Though her step-father, whom she had been fond of, was charged and imprisoned, Martha was certain of and terror-stricken at the prospect of his return. Once she was positive she had sighted him at the mall when shopping with her mother and, in terror, insisted on fleeing the scene. While I could recommend therapy for this child, there are many insults to body and mind that clinical work cannot repair. The capacity to live a reasonable life after such trauma does, however, occur and raises fascinating questions relating to resilience and protective factors in the life outcomes of children. It is to a certain extent because of such resilience that in the world at large, most sexual abuse goes unnoticed, unreported or ignored. Take, for example, Raymond's mother, who brought her son to me, concerned with his academic failure and social ostracism. His loud, strident voice and clumsy, asynchronous gait suggested the random chaos and lack of psychic glue with which some genetically disordered children seem hastily and carelessly assembled by Nature. I saw Raymond only three times. He was eager to avoid all physicians and their products, refusing to return to my office after his third visit.

His mother, who was devoted and competent, came alone in a last session. She had wanted to share with me that Raymond, unbeknownst to him, was conceived in an incestuous relationship between her father, Raymond's grandfather, and herself. Raymond only knew his grandfather as "dad." Her prolonged liaison with her father, free of coercion and enjoyed by both, commenced at age eleven, ending at nineteen. She insisted that the sexual aspect of their relationship stop when she decided to marry a faithful suitor, a decision she consummated when Raymond was two. Both she and her new husband, whose sexual relationship with one another was satisfactory, continued to relate to her father. Raymond, of course, welcomed his grandfather's visits. His mother, who had never sought counseling, described her atypical family ties in a matter-of-fact manner. She somehow accepted her unnatural fate without overt rage or visible shame and had not experienced depression. She felt, in retrospect, exploited but not harmed and was especially proud of her determined emancipation. Raymond's mother was not, in any fundamental way, a troubled woman. There are others like her in this world, some broken, many silently resilient. Raymond was more damaged than his mother, in part by the doubling of recessive genes that contributed to his academic and social impairments.

If we were to imagine Tess's father, Martha's stepfather or Raymond's grandfather in prison, we would see the utter contempt in which those who prey sexually on children are held by their fellow criminals. In the penal code of offenders, pedophilia falls outside the bounds of the acceptable, including rape and murder, markedly decreasing the survival rate of incarcerated child-molesters. Society is more uncertain about the standing of child sexual predators whose numbers are growing and whose age is dropping. Like child murderers, do we diminish the seriousness of their crimes by virtue of their age or prosecute them as adults, fully responsible for their offenses? The genesis of predatory sexuality in pre-pubertal children is complex and entangled with the developmental needs of experimentation and exploration in the service of mastering the bio-psycho-social elements of sexuality. What in the recent past were considered normal "growing pains" now are classified as felonies and prosecuted as such in the very young.

Jack, at fourteen, involved a seven-year-old neighbor in multiple episodes of sexual play including her fellating and masturbating him while he digitally penetrated her vagina. After six or seven episodes, she revealed the details to her mother. I was asked by Jack's attorney to evaluate his status. Jack was a slight, slender youth whose nonchalance, given his circumstances, was striking. While he readily described the interactions with his victim in lurid detail, he expressed no remorse for his actions and had not apologized to the victim or her family. He angered easily, and when wronged by others comfortably entertained homicidal fantasies toward his perceived wrongdoers. I informed Jack, his family and his attorney that he had a serious problem, that it would persist into the future, that he was a risk to others, and that indefinite probation and highly structured treatment were essential to his safekeeping. If self-control is not mastered by four or five years of age, the capacity to delay an impulse remains problematic, often throughout life.

Layton was nine and had already acquired a significant dossier of sexual predation on a younger brother, two neighbor girls and a male peer; he frequently asked classmates if they wanted to have sex with him. This invitation involved his carnal knowledge of fellatio, anal and vaginal intercourse, all of which he had attempted or performed, enjoyed and continued to desire. Layton was big for his age, pale, and made only superficial connections with me during our three meetings. His behavior was ingratiating but unconvincing, making the real Layton, if one existed, hard to find. Flooded well before puberty with sexual desires, he seemed a marginally civilized, amoral boy who had demonstrated to all that he was unsafe in any setting. Like Jack, the history provided by his parents gave me minimal data to unravel the sources of his precocious, indiscriminate, dangerous lust. I urged the school and Layton's family to request state assistance in placing him in a therapeutic, residential program where the danger he posed could be better contained and more intensively explored.

Unlike the sexual arousal and desire in Jack and Layton, childhood eroticism appears in many forms wherein sexuality is secondary to other impulses or needs. The natural exploration of genitals at two or three in toddlers elicits intense sensual pleasure and, when prolonged, relieves depression and anxiety, both of which are biologically suppressed by sexual arousal. The self-soothing, medicinal role of masturbation in the young, particularly in neglected or depressed children, is often stigmatized as sexual abuse; but onanism is Nature's anti-depressant. Similarly, although the homoerotic experimentation of puberty raises flags of alarm, it most often represents efforts to integrate biological sexuality into the self and not molestation. Time, good training and a detailed family and developmental history taken by experienced clinicians are essential tools in separating actual danger from harmless, maturational necessity. They are phenotypes, not genotypes. That is, they look alike but serve altogether different ends. It is also impossible to separate childhood sexuality from the surrounding family process: issues such as interpersonal boundaries, intensity, guiding values, and history of loss may explain what assumes the disguise of excessive sexuality.

Jean was twenty-four when she sought treatment for her depression. A quiet, attractive, seductive young woman, she displayed striking inner impoverishment and emptiness. Such subjective states reliably reflect deprivation of parental care in the first three years of life. Her adolescence had been filled with an endless parade of sexual partners, none of whom seemed emotionally important. Pregnant at twenty, she entered a brief, unhappy marriage that ended shortly after the birth of her now three-year-old daughter. Jean used this charming toddler to overcome her own shyness, much in the same way that the magnetic attraction of puppies generates contact and conversation with strangers. Small talk was otherwise impossible for her. While her family had been intact, a busy father, whose mind was usually elsewhere, and an overwhelmed, irritable mother left Jean and her older brother suffering emotional poverty in the midst of material plenty. Her brother became her main source of company and solace in childhood. Their mutual sexual play began in the years before puberty and was comforting and distracting to both. In adolescence, Jean and her brother became sexual partners, experimenting regularly with oral, anal and genital practices. And while sexual desire was pleasant, for Jean her brother's familiar, soothing physical warmth was primary. His penis in her vagina helped fill her inner vacuum. Her pregnancy was experienced in a similar way as a "fullness" that brought her well-being. But birth was a loss for which she compensated with an endless series of transient sexual contacts that served as analgesics, narcotics, and anti-depressants. During intercourse with these serial, anonymous partners, she fantasized the man's erect penis, as it entered her, as a tiny homunculus of herself. In this way her partner ceased to exist: she related only to herself, repeatedly driven to use the language of sexuality to deal with non-sexual issues of abandonment and neglect that continued to echo in the barren reaches within. Psychotherapy, comforting when present, could not reverse the persistence of her early deprivations. These scars remained, while her therapy ended with my moving out of state to direct the division of Child and Adolescent Psychiatry at the Institute of Living.

Behaviors common to one culture often fare badly or fail when transplanted to another. Nudity, for example, in our country elicits prurient interest while in Northern Europe (and probably most of the world) naked adolescents and adults seem almost clothed. Attitude and custom are powerful garments. So it is with the varieties of sexual practices common to different peoples. But in every land children are intimately involved in sexuality from early in life. There is no single right way to rear our young, sexually or otherwise, and the long term connections between different parenting techniques and life outcomes for our children remain matters of debate. Given this state of our knowledge, or ignorance, it is perhaps wise not to cast the first stone. Dean Rusk, the former Secretary of State, recalling Duhrer's engraving of an all but naked Adam and Eve, warned a war-mongering cabinet "not to lift the fig leaf if you are not prepared to deal with what lies underneath." In child psychiatry one needs to be at ease lifting the fig leaf and dealing with the powerful forces of sexuality that lie beneath.

Chapter Six: Fear and Trembling

Terror in the house does roar." – William Blake

In South Boston ("Southie" to natives) news travels fast. People know what their neighbors are up to and are fiercely loyal to their own. So when the bloody remains of Maggie McGarry's twelve-year-old twin girls were found behind their three-family house on the Monday after Easter, sorrow and alarm hit the streets and the headlines. Kira and Madeline had been raped and bludgeoned to death. There was only one witness, six-year-old Bernard, who was wakened by screams beneath his third-floor window. Peering down on the dimly lit end of his world, Bernard was able to identify, by his long, unruly hair, a sixteen-year-old high school dropout who had been making up to the twins without success. In a rage, he had taken by force what was otherwise denied him. Bernard's statement to the police was sufficiently detailed to charge, arrest, and incarcerate the assailant, whose DNA was present in fingernail scrapings from the girls.

Sui generis, childhood is a time of fear. Nightmares seem real; the storms of raw impulse are violent and often attributed to the outside world, thereby being disowned. *Grimm's Fairy Tales* are indeed grim, accurately reflecting the inner world of children that etches terror onto the ordinary. The benefits of downsizing dread, shrinking reality, are appreciated only later in life. Indeed, the adult world also finds great pleasure in scaring itself, if the success of horror films is indicative. All of this is the known and expected.

But for many children actual horror floods in, at times claiming their spirits, fixing memories and sometimes staining and warping their emerging characters. Certain catastrophes in certain children can forever change biology by creating and maintaining early warning systems, perpetual wariness, in a world that, long afterwards, remains ever hazardous and threatening —in which the demons of nightmares become real. Anna Freud, with her astute clinical eye, observed that children have a finite amount of substance from which to create the self. Children exposed to massive and/or repeated external danger construct an outer, protective "rind" at the expense of an inner world rich in fantasy, imagination and play. Internally such children become, much like Brink's trucks, rigid and constricted. They feel empty. The "Battle Fatigue" of World Wars I and II and, more recently, Post-traumatic Stress are conditions to which children, too, are subject—in wars and natural disasters, on city streets, and sometimes within the frightening privacy of their homes and the bent, corroded circle of family.

I first met Bernard several weeks into the baseball season, and his Red Sox cap assured him choice seating in my office. A pale, slender, reticent boy with a quizzical half-smile, he willingly joined his mother and me. It has often struck me that tragedy frequently cannot be read in the faces of those it assails. The boring rituals of convention sometimes obscure horror and loss. Bernard's receptive manner did not reveal signs of the unnatural disaster that he and his family had just experienced. When a child has been confronted with terrifying danger, the initial therapeutic task is to recreate safety in one small space. That was my goal in the first several, unusually quiet sessions with him. He was drawn to a collection of plastic soldiers in the various poses of war. Play is the equivalent of speech in children. Play in healthy children is scripted by fantasy and imagination. In traumatized children play more often reflects events or experiences that actually happened. Moreover, one sees repetitive play sequences that seem to reflect unconscious efforts to master trauma through its reenactment. A three-year-old girl was referred to me years ago after the wagon she was riding in tumbled into the street in front of an oncoming car. Fear is infectious, and her mother's terror spread to the child, who was clingy, lost bowel control, and wakened at night in alarm. The cure came quickly: again and again she upended a tiny toy wagon in my office, to the accompaniment of the screeching brakes she simulated. Within two weeks her symptoms abated.

Bernard made a fort from Legos and placed one army inside the fort and another assault force outside. There was a lookout post with a window that received special care. A "recon" scout kept careful watch from that site. Bernard did not engage in direct discussion of his sisters' deaths for several weeks. The armies were his voice, the scout his personal narrator. The pyrotechnics and sound effects were chilling, and colleagues in adjacent offices wondered whether Armageddon had found its way to my office. Naturally, the strike force within the fort's four walls was regularly victorious. At times the enemy without took hostages, often two, who were tortured and manhandled by their interrogators. These play sequences closely resembled the murder of Bernard's sisters. I waited for my openings. Bernard permitted me to play the well-positioned scout. I commented on the dangers about, the soldiers' vulnerability, the terror of an ambush, the need for medics, and the burial of the war dead on both sides.

According to his mother, Bernard had abandoned friends. She herself was overwhelmed by sorrow, further straining Bernard's supports. I told my wife that I imagined bringing him home, adopting him. It was a fantasy, of course, my response to his needs. If I count the number of children waiting in line for my family's care over the years, it would put Mia Farrow and Angelina Jolie to shame. Gradually, over the weeks of summer and fall, Bernard began to draw pictures of his house and the crime scene. His words were spare, addressing his dread in watching his sisters die. He visited their grave once weekly with his mother and began to weep at the graveside. The newspapers covered the case and the forthcoming trial. Bernard's anxiety rose again, since he wondered if the murderer would come after him for being a *stoolie*. "What if he breaks out of jail? He knows my house, and our dog never barks at strangers. Or maybe he'll get a friend to take me out." It was hard to reassure him that his fears were groundless. For the rest of his life, I supposed, no fears would be groundless for Bernard.

Tentatively, haltingly at first, after many weeks we began to assemble the jagged fragments of Bernard's life. His dreams re-played the murders but woke him less often. I had the impression that this disaster was becoming encapsulated, like an abscess, but I knew better than to lance it now. There would be ample time for further drainage in the years to come. He began bringing in the sports page to discuss the prospects for the Sox. He sought the company of friends he had avoided for a time, and his schoolwork improved. The trial court awarded Bernard substantial monies for future psychotherapy.

When Bernard was referred to me I welcomed the opportunity to help him and his family recreate their shattered universe. I knew that I was revisiting a sad land unfortunately known to me since the death of my second son, Nicholas. Nicholas was riding his bike during a family vacation in France when he was hit by a car. He died several hours later. There were moments in the work with Bernard and his family, and with many other patients in similar straits, none of whom knew of my son's death, when my own sorrow and memories surfaced. Surely I was mastering my trauma as well as theirs. I knew of a child's bloody, broken body, of unspeakable horror, futile rage at the missing, the silence louder than the noise of life, and the empty, shadowy inner theater where, without audience and unknown to the outside world, a distracting documentary runs night and day. In such instances as Bernard's, I help and am helped; but I am very careful, as anyone in similar circumstances needs to be, to maintain the professional boundary that allows me, by virtue of my own experiences, to better serve my patients. They are not there to serve me. The use of my pain is respect for and remembrance of the dead. My *yahrzeit* for Nicholas.

Maria, a plump, loud, unruly six-year-old with hair akimbo, was seen once during a hospital inpatient consultation. She was referred to the unit after threatening her infant brother with a kitchen knife. Brutal, impulsive violence was the lullaby of her early years: her mother was beaten regularly by a succession of drunken, explosive men whose tantrums Maria feared and hated. In hospital she only permitted female staff to touch or approach, watchfully avoiding the company of men. Her nights were full of agitation and, according to staff, she rarely slept, hyper-alert and startled by the slightest ambient sounds. I was asked to evaluate this state of eternal arousal, this internal, summer Lapland where night is day and sleep denied.

I could approach Maria only as she sat on the lap of a nurse she had befriended. She vocally protested my presence and assured me with blazing eyes that she would not talk, would not utter a word, and to demonstrate her determination pursed her lips into a hard, straight, bloodless line of grim defiance. In such situations I have learned to practice, in memory of Gary Cooper, a dialogue that is a monologue requiring no answers. Puzzled by my enthusiastic support of her silence, Maria occasionally glanced at me furtively. I began narrating the life of a child I knew who was always upset, a girl just her age who was always frightened by the loud noise of fights in her house.

Maria could not resist and asked if it was someone she knew. This *doppelganger*, I went on, was always scared and very angry that her mommy did not protect her from such chaos. Maria nodded. And, I added, many times she wanted to run away and find a mother who really loved her. Maria turned to her nurse and whispered, "I run away a lot," then sank farther into the soft, ample cushion of her caregiver's lap. I shared with Maria, avoiding her gaze, that this child needed to know that she was safe, that her mommy was safe, and that even six-year-olds can dial 911. With this apparently novel advice, Maria's eyelids began to droop. The police, I reminded her, were ready night and day, waiting to protect little girls and carry off noisy, dangerous men. And did she know any lady police? They were just as strong as the men. Maria, barely nodding, fell into a peaceful sleep, her body's taut cables uncoiling for the first time. I hoped she was dreaming of a career in public safety; it is never too early to plant the seeds of a vocation, of competence and self-respect that may transform the open wounds of trauma into a viable future.

Post-traumatic Stress Disorder has become lucrative. Many lawsuits are considered or initiated with the intent to prove psychological damages resulting from calamities of one sort or another that a generation ago would have been taken as the luck of the draw: auto accidents, predatory teachers and circumcisions that go awry. In children especially, the prediction of future damages becomes relevant but murky. Hippocrates was not a fortune-teller. And Nature not infrequently confounds clinicians as well as meteorologists, welcome proof that mankind controls less than it thinks. Child and adolescent psychiatrists are often asked to become experts in such cases. Humility, integrity, thoroughness and a sense of humor are paramount to practitioners who enter these lists. Fondness for chess and detective work are also helpful.

Particularly fascinating to me are the children who do not develop symptoms when exposed to the same events as their afflicted peers. This hopeful puzzle, for it speaks to resilience, is especially evident in evaluating groups of children in identical circumstances. A school board rightfully besieged by worried and irate parents asked me to interview ten female adolescents molested by a troubled janitor four years earlier. Five of these young women, despite vivid memories of clear abuse, were spirited teens, free of post-traumatic stigmata, and eager to share with me their academic, social or athletic success. Others were plagued by agonizing shyness, shame about their bodies, nightmares recalling the experience and intrusive, disturbing "flashbacks." Two had neither memories nor detectable *sequelae* and were optimistic about the future. The melodramatic, extravagant claims of one girl were simply not credible. These varied outcomes are characteristic of responses to major stressors and underscore the importance of protective factors in determining whether any one child will succumb to trauma.

There are some children who, finding themselves in sudden, terrifying or even life-threatening circumstances, show few if any overt signs of trouble until months or years later when a hidden memory rises to consciousness, often prodded by a sight, sound or setting linked to the original trauma. Willie, a thirteen-year-old little league ace, was an outstanding student, good friend and seemingly solid boy. Everyone praised him. He loved animals and at age nine had played with a neighbor's dog in his backyard. Without warning the dog had turned on Willie, attacking him viciously, lacerating his face and dragging him to the ground. Only a passing motorist's rescue efforts freed Willie, who then went by ambulance to the hospital. Several surgeries were required to repair the damage. Willie's life did not change much thereafter; his supportive and unflappable parents helped their son through this crisis with their steady ways. Four years later Willie happened on a dog resembling the attacker in a similar setting and became acutely depressed. Flashbacks of the original incident flooded his mind and the isolated phrase "I will die" floated in and out of his awareness, always accompanied by terror and despair. He recalled that this grim prediction had silently possessed him as he rode to the hospital after the dog's attack. Psychotherapy was strongly recommended to bring peace to this thoughtful, sensitive, fundamentally healthy boy.

Bill Sack, a colleague and good friend, has studied the adjustment of adolescent Cambodian immigrants to this country over the past twenty years. All of these youths witnessed carnage, torture, the killing of friends and family, and the destruction of their homes. They left their country to enter a new, strange land without the benefits of a familiar language, familiar landscape, or friends. Like the survivors of other Holocausts, their memories are shards of pain that tear, continuously and without warning, through the fabric of the ordinary, prompted by a sight, a sound, a smell, a taste. Without the ordinary we can neither assemble nor reassemble our lives. But many of these youths move forward, becoming successful students, entrepreneurs, professionals and even politicians. Their minds remain beleaguered by flashbacks of horror that run simultaneously and in parallel with hopefulness, will and the mastery of new tasks. Those who not only survive but prevail over the horror of their earlier lives have in common the reliable presence, through the turmoil, of one loving, devoted adult: a necessary and sufficient condition to live tolerably in the presence of pain while addressing the needs of present and future. One loving adult helps the eye stay focused not on what was but on what is or is yet to come.

While trauma may atrophy, loosen its grip on the mind, with and sometimes without therapeutic help, there are situations in childhood where that grip tightens and expands. In these cases it becomes difficult for the clinician to differentiate the flashbacks of post-traumatic stress from the hallucinations of psychosis. I have wondered, in fact, whether in some situations the discontinuous, episodic flashbacks of trauma become increasingly fixed and, when finally immobile, come to rest in the form of madness. I once interviewed a twelve-year-old girl, Abbey, in a diagnostic seminar. A flushed, sweaty, pallid youngster, she appeared terrified of unidentified dangers, entering the interviewing room as a camera, scanning every face, every object of furniture and every door before seating herself near me.

As I learned about Abbey's life, she alleged that an older brother had repeatedly raped her over several years. As she haltingly recounted this horror, she glanced in all directions, groaning and wringing her hands; her eyes finally lighted upon a cabinet of dark wood at which she stared intently with mounting dread. "There he is, there he is again, oh no, no, no." Calming after some minutes, Abbey was able to describe the image of her brother's face glaring at her, menacing her, on the cabinet door in much the same manner that the face of Jacob Marley appeared to Scrooge on the knocker of his front entrance. These apparitions were more or less constant for Abbey, pursuing her in any place at any time. Her dread and dysfunction were of such proportions as to bring her daily life to a halt. In effect, she was psychotic without the fully expressed stigmata of psychosis. Just as a recurrent, obsessional thought, such as a hypochondriacal concern, can merge into the delusional, becoming fact rather than fancy, so it was with Abbey's visions of her brother. What then is mental illness? Whence does it come, inside out or outside in? Is it possible to observe the birth and life of madness in the laboratory of trauma—to see outer events enter the mind and brain, not just as memories but as larger, more malignant presences that metastasize to all corners of being? These questions, like the work that prompts them, display a terrible beauty.

The admonition of Sophocles, "Count no man fortunate until the day he dies," seems wisely to acknowledge the inevitability of misfortune throughout the course of life. That every man comes, sooner or later, face to face with horror is all too true. Most such events go unreported and, sometimes, unnoticed. But when these confrontations take place in childhood their volume is louder, the space they occupy larger, and their insinuation into the developing self more profound. Whether affected by single events, or years of exposure as in wars or urban ghetto life, the course of an afflicted child's life veers and recovers, or falls off the track of development. Child psychiatrists can sometimes provide a road map, without shortcuts, toward the resumption of travel in the right direction. I have come to see that the presence or persistence of post-traumatic symptoms need not outweigh the healthy capacity to live. One can live, even well, with horror if it is managed, contained or kept at bay. Health matters, illness sometimes does not. We can walk on one leg, see with one eye, write with one hand despite the fates. The soul, not the body, needs symmetry.

CHAPTER SEVEN: ROOTED SORROWS

What cannot be said will get wept. – Sappho

Meryl was driving, her new baby on her lap; suddenly, out of control, the car careened wildly down a bleak, unlit, unfamiliar street. Running the curb, it smashed violently into the wall surrounding a more familiar house. At the moment of impact Meryl and the baby fused, became one, and were thrown to the sidewalk, lying supine, alone. No help came. In time, a newsman, expressionless, looked down on her, shot camera footage and, departing with neither greeting nor good-bye, left the still unattended Meryl in gray, shadowy silence. She wakened from her dream in hopelessness and despair, the same emotions that led her to seek consultation. I shivered at the creative elegance, the beauty of this dream that had come to light like an author's lost manuscript, revealing previously unknown chapters of a life. Meryl, a Rubenesque mother of two, had kept company with depression in her earliest memories. She could not recall a time when she'd been free of gloom. Since the birth of her last child, now five months old, her mood had darkened. She ruminated about suicide in the midst of a major post-partum depression. Her dream suggested to me that the birth of her second child had activated memories of despair from the time of her own birth. The robotic newsman might have been a stand-in for an unresponsive, depressed parent whose inability to provide care left Meryl depressed from infancy.

She approached her father, who confirmed a family secret: his wife had required a three-month psychiatric hospitalization after Meryl's arrival and was marginally functional for most of her daughter's first year. Anna Freud observed that infants in this situation "follow their mothers into depression," taking in the mood itself as milk, even if soured. All that is available to them as sustenance is their mother's despair. In later life this bad meal can present itself as chronic depression that is often untreatable. Though mother (deep within) is black and bleak, her child holds on to her for dear life: she is all of the known world. Meryl's dream was an accurate chronicle of her beginnings in the grip of her mother's melancholy. Unexpectedly, she responded well to anti-depressant medication. Within a month her mood lightened and she was better able to survive the rigors of new parenthood. She interrupted her treatment, relieved and grateful.

Historically, the initial descriptions of depression in child psychiatry were limited to the severe, maternal-deprivation syndromes of infancy, Marasmus and "failure to thrive," which lead infants to withdraw, refuse food, lose weight, stop growing, and often die. Meryl was fortunate: we have come a long way toward overcoming our Victorian legacy of childhood as a blissful time, a legacy that has provided added fuel for a skeptical public that doubts the possibility that young children can suffer depression. At the time of my training in the Sixties, the modest literature on childhood mood disorders was speculative and unconvincing. What presumably did not exist in our patients was neither looked for nor seen. I recall my disbelief at the suicide of a high school classmate, a tragic event for which I could find no frame of reference. Only in the last twenty-five years has clinical and biological research described and documented the relatively high prevalence of mood disorders in childhood and adolescence, their genetic and familial basis, and their response to psychotherapies and anti-depressants. Ten to fifteen percent of randomly surveyed elementary and middle school students have thought about suicide. It is particularly poignant to witness the pain of despair in the young where it feels, somehow, more out of place, more intense and desperate than in adults or the elderly. I am especially moved by such moods in children.

The onset of depression prior to puberty, unless it is clearly situational, unfortunately increases the likelihood of mood disorders in adolescence and adult life. Meryl's story was typical of this pattern. I feel some urgency to reverse depression in this early onset population, hoping to change a child's odds for the better. In this quest, a child's character is a potent force that can help overcome a discouraging prognosis.

I was asked to see Francie, then eight, on an inpatient basis. She had been admitted after seriously assaulting a third grade classmate whom she felt had insulted her. For the month prior to this assault she slept poorly, sometimes unable to fall asleep until three or four in the morning, pacing her house while banging kitchen pots together in a noisy, maddening, one-person parade. Her parents had recently divorced. There was a history of alcoholism, serious gambling and Bipolar Disorder in the family. While the diagnosis of manic depression in pre-pubertal children is rare, Francie had enough stigmata to suggest that disorder. By the time I saw her, she had terrorized the other children on the unit and, as a cyclone of activity, was beginning to wear on a usually patient staff.

She welcomed me with contempt: "You bald, ugly, stupid little man." I could not resist smiling at this scornful greeting, launching Francie into a tirade of further derisive commentary on my dress, my big nose and my credentials. Had she been an adult, her words would not have entertained me, but coming out of a child's mouth they seemed incongruous and harmless. In fact, I admired her spunk and her pride, and saw that her eyes were warmer than her words. I liked her, admired her, respected her candor and continued to do so through the years of our work together. She was bright, pretty, enormously stubborn, and like most bipolar children, she was intensely, perpetually irritable. "I could kill you," she warned me, "I could kill myself." This was my first glance at the hopelessness and futility that would plague Francie as she sank, through the years, into prolonged periods of suicidal gloom. Her parents seemed to trust me, and I agreed to take her on as a patient. In some way I was hopeful about this child.

Bipolar children require a delicate balance of medications that are potentially toxic and dangerous. Mood stabilizers such as lithium, Depakote or the newer agents must be employed to level the turmoil of mania, insulate the bare wires of the mind. Anti-depressants raise the bar on despair but can provoke mania; the side effect of weight gain is especially troublesome to girls, who impulsively stop their medication if their bodies begin to change. As bipolar children grow in size and age, a previously stable regimen loses its effectiveness and new combinations must be tried. Adolescence does not thrive on sickness or its cure. Non-compliance with medication is the rule, the consequences of which in Bipolar Disorder are always serious. Francie and her mother, with whom she lived, were remarkably tolerant of my pharmaceutical juggling, though my patient could not resist a complimentary "You don't know what you're doing Dr. R; I may need an expert."

Through elementary and middle school, and then into high school, Francie struggled to keep her agitated, overly busy mind on learning while trying to enter a social world that was put off by her blunt, hurtful rudeness and chronic, defensive disdain. Her only friends, at times, were her guidance counselors. She was determined to join but didn't know the steps of the dance. I often felt that my office was kind of a refueling stop, a place for her to renew her determination. We had become good friends. She became calmer, less feisty and increasingly respectful. In despair, on one occasion, Francie asked, "What really is wrong with me?" She knew, of course, that she had been called bipolar but had been too scared to explore the meaning of that word. I drew a bell-shaped curve on paper to illustrate the universality of all traits and behaviors and reviewed with her the population curve of bipolar traits. We talked of racing thoughts, mood instability and irritability. We discussed the balancing actions of the mood stabilizers and anti-depressants. Francie asked to keep the sketch. I added, "You are not bipolar, you are not this illness: you are yourself and always will be. The bipolar condition, like a birthmark, is part of you but is not who you are, what matters to you, or how you choose to live your life. If you had diabetes it would not be you either." She understood what I wanted her to grasp, and she knew that I meant it. She smiled.

When Francie reached her junior year in high school, she underwent a change that I did not, do not understand. At the age when bipolar conditions often become more severe, her moods became more even, her irritability diminished, and her deep depressions virtually disappeared. She had previously worn her hair long, often covering her face. Now she had it cut as to reveal her natural beauty. The lines of her face became sharp, well defined; the crystallization of self within was evident without. On her own initiative, without leads or connections, this socially clumsy young woman found an excellent job. Francie was courageous; she did not complain about her illness and resisted shame after her multiple hospitalizations. She was tough enough, sufficiently self-respecting, not to allow herself, or others, to identify her as different or "crazy." And while she was at times eccentric, old beyond her years, she had developed antibodies to adversity through overcoming it. There are heroes on a small scale. Francie qualified.

The almost imperceptible physical signs in Francie that heralded change are reliable clues in all assessments of patients. In addition to skin turgor and color, posture, gait, dress, hygiene, tone of voice, brightness of gaze, and eye contact are especially informative. Progress in therapy is more accurately measured by these silent, external signals than by the noise of words. In most instances the body, unlike the tongue, seems incapable of deception. The eyes have it. And in depression the body frequently becomes the repository of woes that are of the spirit, not the flesh. The milder end of this spectrum is hypochondriasis; the more severe depressions may present themselves as somatic delusions, convictions that the body is rotting, organs shrinking, teeth falling out, fatal illness developing.

Sandra was orphaned at eight when her parents were killed in a highway accident. After this tragedy she was raised by her maternal grandmother. At age fourteen Sandra's grandmother developed stomach pains that were diagnosed as a gastric malignancy. She died a pain-filled death six months later. Two months after this loss, Sandra was hospitalized in a state of disorganization. A gaunt, homely girl with facial acne, she was almost mute. She refused food, already looking wasted and ill. She sat doubled over, clutching her stomach, grimacing and moaning as if in pain. I sat with her, and while she made eye contact, she did not speak. I carried on a monologue: "You miss your grandmother (her groaning intensifies). It is so sad to lose her, you must feel all alone (she doubles over). You're worried that you have stomach cancer (she meets my eyes) but the doctor says you're fine. You're trying to keep your grandmother inside (load groan), you want to be with her." Our meetings for a time were iterations of each other, my commentary interrupted periodically by the vivid body English of Sandra's responses. Freud's classic paper, "Mourning and Melancholia," described Sandra's dynamics: to deal with the loss of a loved one, the bereaved incorporates that person, symptoms and all, taking them in wholesale, living and dead symbolically fusing, with the specific symptoms from which the loved one died most prominent in the somatic display.

Sandra began lingering, wraith-like, by my office door, a beseeching look crossing her face whenever I came into view. Shortly she began wailing, almost keening, in a plaintive whine, "Dr. Robson, help me, please help me." As her verbal output increased, her somatic behavior diminished. She moved out of her body, back to her mind when the unbearable pain of this death began to be more tolerable. She wept in paroxysms of grief interspersed with fury at all of the loved ones who had abandoned her, now appearing clinically depressed but vocal, organized and able to eat again. I wondered how she could live, what sustained her in the face of her ill-fated life. I experienced her stark, overwhelming grief and wept with her. Finally, she was discharged to the home of a relative in another city. Some of life's injuries are too severe to heal, leaving the patient crippled or deformed. Within, Sandra's landscape had become as barren and charred as Dresden after the bombing; her stomach's aching ceased, but I'm certain she continued to live in pain.

To an adolescent, time is boundless; when one hurts it seems the pain will never stop. In such circumstances suicide becomes a cure, a drastic, irreversible analgesic. For the child psychiatrist the risk of self-destruction is ever-present; it hovers over every clinical situation where depression is prominent and requires diligent monitoring, though it is an option one would rather forget. Suicides in adults usually involve lengthy planning and careful implementation; in adolescence impulsive acts are more the rule. Available pills, car keys, or a gun, when the family is out of the home at a time of anguish, are sufficient to bring on sudden, unexpected death. Darren was different.

In adolescent suicides, one often finds a prior history of depression. Darren began drinking at twelve. He liked the taste of alcohol, and by sixteen, when I had brief contact with him, was an alcoholic. His father, absent in Darren's life since infancy, was also alcohol-addicted and prone to major depressive episodes. Alcohol and depression are genetic and familial companions living in the same dangerous biological dwelling. Darren's grades had been declining precipitously following a break-up with a girlfriend with whom he had been closely but stormily involved for the preceding two years. On the day prior to his hospitalization, Darren began drinking, alone, in the afternoon. Out of liquor, he drove to the nearest package store, where he was well known, purchased a fifth of cheap whiskey and, in the darkness of evening, began to drink it behind the store. He consumed the entire bottle, lost consciousness, and was virtually invisible to all who passed. The local police, who frequented this store, happened by chance to pull in far enough to see Darren's prostrate body some twelve hours later. He remained in coma after his hospitalization, near death from alcohol poisoning. When he was sufficiently recovered to talk, I was asked to evaluate the risk of suicide and recommend a plan of treatment.

This six-foot-plus, two-hundred-pounder looked older than his years; he resembled a college-age defensive lineman. His voice was slow, deep and monotonic, his eyes dull, his emotional expression flat and muted, his thinking labored. As with many males, Darren's conscious wish to die was shared with no one and his suicidal act was deliberately carried out in isolation, increasing the likelihood of death and minimizing the possibility of rescue. A girl of that age would probably have shared her despair with someone and would, in all likelihood, have located herself where she would be found. The social skills and impulses of girls decrease the danger of their suicide attempts, though they make many more than males.

Like the lost man unwilling to ask for directions, Darren surrounded himself with lethal silence. He resented his salvation, convinced that the gray, painless obscurity of death was a right taken unjustly from him. He was clear, matter of fact with me regarding his continuing intention to end life; there were no qualifiers. I always ask depressed children and teens the color of their mood. Black is a poor sign, the hue of hopelessness and Darren's selection. I also ask what a child loves and is good at, convinced that competence at even one thing can strengthen if not save a life. Darren answered: "Nothing, I'm good at nothing, not even dying." When the risk is high I feel scared. I was scared in Darren's case and, against his will, committed him to ongoing inpatient care. But the wish to die, when unambiguous, is a determined ambition not to be thwarted. Darren's compass pointed in only one grim direction. There were no forks in the road ahead.

For many suicidal teens, Darren's Ahab-like single-mindedness is absent. The act is more impulsive, and while it may succeed, at times by mistake, life is still valued. I have become, however, increasingly concerned that suicide is an ever more acceptable choice to the young adult at this time in history. And the value of life, sometimes taken for a pair of Air Jordans, has steadily declined. The erosion of family structure, the dilution of values by which to live, media exposure, and the ready availability of weapons contribute to the adolescent suicide rate. But the tragedy of a wasted young life, whether compromised by untreated mood disorders or ended by death, lies not in the hands of chance. It is avoidable. There are ample hammer blows of misfortune that one cannot easily sidestep. But to willingly step into their path squanders opportunity. It mocks life. The birds I most love, the Red-tail Hawk and Great Blue Heron, do not mock and never squander. My Dachshund, Isabella, cannot be dissuaded from love or life or joy. I bring her to my office.

Nowhere has the beauty and elegance of the mind been more apparent to me than in the unfolding of mourning in a depressed sixteen-year-old girl whose estranged, troubled father had killed her mother and himself while Alyssa was at school. She was referred to me by her principal. Alyssa was a short, muscular young woman with a boyish build and a boyish look topped with short-cut red hair. Her initial response included, much to her chagrin, sudden fantasies of killing friends with whom she might be chatting in the hall between classes. These violent shorts were, she said, altogether out of character for her, and frightening. Her thoughts at bedtime scattered in all directions and her sleep was troubled by terrifying dreams. She assured me that her parents' death was "not a problem." When the pot is about to boil over, you do not turn up the heat. I prescribed a low dose of a major tranquilizer, and the frequency and intensity of Alyssa's horror films diminished. I suggested to her that they were "decoys," distracting her from her sorrow and pain.

Shortly these terrifying images were replaced by the sound of a woman's voice weeping uncontrollably. This experience occurred at random times and initially was as frightening as the earlier fantasies. "Alyssa," I asked, "whose voice, whose pain do you think that is?" "Nobody I know," she answered. I suggested that her mind was playing kindly tricks, keeping her grief at arm's length, waiting for a stronger, better time to mourn with her own voice, her own tears. "Will that come out of the blue?" she asked. Knowing that it might, I gave her my cell phone number and made certain that she felt comfortable calling me at any time of night or day. Two weeks later Alyssa reported that she rarely heard the sorrowful voice but now was having "weird" dreams. In one that was particularly distressing, her younger sister was sitting on her lap, sobbing and wanting to be held and hugged. "You're passing the buck," I joked. "Your sister has her own therapist and her needs are being met." Alyssa was very bright and, psychologically speaking, a quick study. "I get it, I get it," she exclaimed, "it's a switcheroo." "Yep," I answered, "and you're about ready to call a spade a spade."

She was, and in time the tragedy of her life became bearable through her own tears, her own sorrow, her own undisguised pain. Her mind's kindly choreographer was expert in timing and design, never asking more of her charge than she could bear. Such is the artistry of the unconscious drama coach we carry within.

My training in child psychiatry was woefully impoverished in biological approaches to diagnosis and treatment. Of course, few of the array of currently available medications and the research studies to test their efficacy had made their appearance. My practice over the last twenty years has involved many patients needing pharmacotherapy in addition to counseling. While biology is not my native tongue, the advent of medications that address the conditions that I regularly encounter has brought me closer to my identity as a physician. Unlike some of my colleagues, I find a particular sense of competence in properly medicating children and adolescents. The results are sometimes dramatic and gratifying. Archaic Greek won't buy you breakfast in modern Athens.

Depression is a universal experience. The parent who says to a child in pain, "Buck up, you don't have it so bad" needs a short course in remembering. For the child with a blackly depressive mood, more tools than time's passage are required: psychotherapy, medication and a panoramic lens that widens one's view of the world. My favorite metaphor with children who have abandoned all hope is the inevitable batting slump that topflight major league hitters suffer, usually more than once in the course of a season. They avoid despair by focusing on what they can correct before coming to the plate again, increasing the chances of better luck next time. Will doesn't always produce a way, but it helps when hell waits around one's corner.

CHAPTER EIGHT: VISITATIONS

One trembles to think of that mysterious thing in the soul,
which seems to acknowledge no human jurisdiction, but in
spite of the individual's own innocent self, will still dream hor-
rid dreams, and mention unmentionable thoughts.

– Herman Melville

The torments of Hell were not merely scriptural in me-
dieval times; obsessive thoughts and compulsive acts
plagued the early clerics as visitations of the Devil himself. It
was commonplace that during the performance of the Mass,
practitioners suddenly and repeatedly visualized Christ squat-
ting and defecating on the altar, a profane image that filled its
owner with shame and disgust and could come from nowhere
but the darker regions. Before Freud linked obsessions to emotional states such as aggression, sexuality or guilt, and the later
insights of biological psychiatry began to trace and treat their
neurochemistry, virtually nothing was known of the origins
of these phenomena. But superstition and rituals to ward off
calamity were as familiar to Sophocles as they are to children,
as seen in their games, and to major league baseball players.
Generations of (not so innocent) schoolchildren have carefully side-stepped the crack in a sidewalk to spare their mothers
a broken back.

All varieties of psychological disorder, beginning in childhood
and moving into adolescence and adult life, tend to be organized by obsessive-compulsive phenomena, whether they are
repetitive images or ritualized behaviors. In this respect they
may alert the clinician, like highway flares, to trouble ahead.
At times they are furtive, arriving suddenly and silently, leav-

ing without a trace. Or they may become relatively fixed as annoying companions or alien, persecutory furies. A scholar in this field tries to comfort his troubled patients by thinking of their obsessional images as "mind-farts," random, harmless flatus that passes. But children so afflicted need more than Tums for comfort.

Obsessive-compulsive phenomena conform to a bell-shaped curve, one end of which resembles normal variants. In toddlers and preschoolers, for example, one can observe a variety of such behaviors; usually they generate a smile or an anecdote and pass out of the child's repertoire and the parent's awareness. I have watched one-year-old infants carefully, systematically pluck bits of food or dust from their clothing, upset if they are unable to do so immediately. Toddlers may organize their toys in a particular manner that neither they nor an adult can alter without a tantrum. For most young children these ritualistic habits are of no developmental consequence; they are epiphenomena and harmless add-ons. In others they take on greater significance.

Carolee was four when she went to live with her paternal grandmother. Born in a trailer park, witness to sexual orgies and parental violence, she lacked the filters to screen out the toxins of those early years. She fought off intrusive memory with an array of repetitive eccentricities. This plump, appealing preschooler with long, strawberry blonde hair, was wide-eyed and wary. A tiny martinet, she dominated her grandmother, whom she had in tow when I first met her. "No, Gram, I won't talk to him, I don't like him, I won't go in there." To my friendly greeting, she responded "No." I said nothing, walked into my office, took out the dolls and dollhouse and, sitting on the floor, began my solitary play; I did not look at Carolee, who shortly clambered down beside me, eyeing the house and me alternately. I continued furnishing the dollhouse without glancing at her, enticing her with delicious neglect she succumbed to. Soon we were playing together. "It's safe in this house," I murmured. Her precocious language development was helpful as we moved between actions and words.

At home, Carolee's tyrannical rituals disrupted the household from morning to night. Her food preferences were limited to cranberry juice and canned baby peas, which she ate one at a time, pinched between her right thumb and forefinger. The peas had to make a circle that Carolee traversed from left to right; any violation of this sequence required going back to the beginning, amidst much distress. Dressing was worse, her acceptable selections limited to pink, flowered dresses with white hems. Bedtime, for frightened children the precursor to dark, solitary outer space, was interminable. Grandmother had to sit with arms folded and legs crossed; three dolls were placed in the same spots to guard Carolee as her hair was brushed until it was free of all asymmetries. The same prayer, in the same tone of voice and volume, was uttered repetitively until grandmother got it right, exactly right. If she survived the night without terror, the morning perturbations were almost comical. Carolee, never schooled in dance, insisted on twirling three times, like a miniature ballerina, to ward off some evil presence as she climbed down from her bed; these gyrations made her dizzy enough that she lurched unsteadily to the bathroom, where new ceremonies were conducted.

My visits with Carolee were limited to managing her regimen of medications; I saw her perhaps three or four times a year over several years, but we had a good connection. When she saw me coming to greet her in the waiting room, she smiled broadly, darting into my office to pull out familiar toys. Her rituals decreased but remained, and when she was anxious, as in school, they intensified. She was a shy child, and odd enough to make peer relations complicated. I could imagine her in twenty years as a dedicated, quirky, reference librarian.

Compulsions like Carolee's are visible to the world at large, while obsessive thoughts are the private property of each owner, an unhappy audience of one. Only when the content or frequency of such mental tics becomes painful or excessive are they exposed to the light of day. Allie sat sullenly in my waiting room. At eight, she was unusually short, her freckles and tousled jet-black hair making her appear younger than her years. The oldest child of Boston Brahmins, her privileged life had not brought her joy. She rarely smiled, presenting a dour mien in keeping with the bedtime bouts of despair that her parents described: abject, miserable, she would loudly bewail her unhappy lot with, "I hate my life, I hate my family, I'd be better off dead," or "This is the worst day of my life." These tearful, heartfelt diatribes alarmed her parents, who could discover no cause for such gloom. It was entirely out of keeping with her many gifts: a sharp intellect, athletic prowess, artistic competence and a very wry sense of humor. None of these kept Allie from feeling "ugly, really ugly." She had given me my opening.

We had become friends. What, I wondered with Allie, was this "ugly" business in a pretty, smart girl like her? Sheepishly, she answered, "my bad thoughts, my troubles." She was silent, squirming. "Can you draw them for me?" I asked. "You know my drawings stink...you can't help me," she said bitterly, accusatorily. No one can help me." And she wept, refusing my efforts to comfort her. I told Allie that I used to see a boy her age who brought me his arsenal of "bad thoughts," sadistic fantasies involving tearing family members limb from limb, urinating on his new baby brother, and more. She brightened and listened intently. When I was done, she asked where he lived, what he looked like, and whether he attended her school. She thought she knew him. Hadn't she seen him in my waiting room last week? Then she offered, "Do you want to hear about mine?" I gave an uninterestrd shrug impossible to resist, and her unburdening began.

There were three distinct and powerful obsessions: one involved her front teeth and gums being torn from her mouth (she rubbed her mouth and grimaced in the telling); a second image displayed both wrists bleeding, punctured by a sharp object. Only in time was the third described: the fingernails of her right hand, with which she masturbated as a sedative during sleepless nights, being torn off one by one. For Allie these imaginative events were concrete, physical realities. "You know," I offered, "those are just thoughts; they seem real but they are just feelings like everyone has. You feel bad when you tickle yourself, but losing your fingernails, that's a little much. Why not take number three as a signal you are feeling naughty, naughtier than you are?" As together we translated, broke the code of these images, Allie wrote out agendas prior to our meetings to focus the work, arriving weekly with a yellow sheet with issues written out in order, a list of psychological errands.

Her nocturnal implosions diminished, but her depression continued and her self-loathing remained. For now we focused our attention on the harsh, cruel tenor of her intolerant conscience and the fury she often felt over perceived slights: girlfriends she envied or teachers who awarded her less than perfect grades. But new obsessions were born over the years of our therapy. By eleven, Allie had developed modest breast buds; shortly after being teased about their diminutive size she developed a repetitive image and painful sensation of both breasts being pierced by a knife. The meaning of this obsession became, without prompting, immediately clear to Allie, who observed, "My troubles have to do with what I don't like about myself." Her capacity to reflect on an important dynamic of her thoughts allowed me to comment: "So think of them all as poems or messages that can be put into words like you did just now, harmless poems, symbols that are simply pictures of feelings."

Allie's mood improved but her obsessive thoughts, while bothering her less, did not decrease in frequency. Allie, her parents and I agreed upon a trial of Fluvoxamine, a medication helpful in the management of Allie's disorder. Within a month there was a notable decrease in all of her thoughts and a greater ability to disregard them. Rectal bleeding forced Allie to undergo a colonoscopy; this intrusive procedure was not only an assault but, naturally, carried a sexual meaning to a pubertal girl. For Allie it was a physically painful procedure. Some weeks thereafter she reported an obsession involving a painful piercing of her anus, a sequence she was now familiar with and could translate with relative ease. Then, opening a session, she described a curative dream: she was alone in a dark, Hitchcock-like house with male intruders threatening at the windows. Friends appeared and plotted with her to give the assailants laxatives, a part of her prepping for the colonoscopy she found especially unpleasant. She had dreamed for her enemies a proper but harmless revenge, a taste of their own medicine. Her dream was about mastery and health: friends joining her to convert the helpless status of patient into one of active, collaborative problem-solving. It was also funny, and when she reviewed it with me I burst out laughing, much to Allie's delight. Her dream reflected age-appropriate, mature perspective that to me was encouraging.

By the time she reached thirteen, Allie's obsessions had receded. They had either disappeared from view or, when visible, had faded to irrelevant wallpaper that rarely claimed her attention or distressed her. She wondered if they might never disappear entirely. Because they did not deter the healthy progress of her development they loomed small to both Allie and me. She experienced depression from time to time around the same issues with which she had begun: remaining hypersensitive to rejection, prone to envy others and, and quick to criticize her basically loving family. But she moved away from black and white, all or none, introducing increasing amounts of gray onto her palette. The greater part of her energies was directed at academic success, social comfort with friends, and a willingness to try new activities and master them. She was seen as a leader by her peers. The swarm of boys who hovered around her tended to dismiss her feelings of unattractiveness. Her core was solid and she steadily amassed new skills that built upon one another. She continued to see me, musing from time to time on a career in child psychiatry, using me increasingly as a mentor. She knew that I genuinely believed in her strength and her prospects for a rich and productive life. On one occasion I told Allie that someday her "troubles" might be of use to her, that what are liabilities at one time in life may become assets at another, that enemies can become friends. "They are just poems; poems are not only about beautiful things," I reminded her, "just poems that need reading." Allie was last seen when she was eighteen; she was in college and enjoying both academics and social life. Her obsessions seemed dimmer and less disruptive to her being.

In some children lacking Allie's strengths, the self seems organized, held together, by a fragile assemblage of rituals, behind which lies psychological chaos. Rituals in such situations represent the last vestige of an orderly universe. Nan seemed to like animals more than people. She was at ease with all the creatures of the field. I saw her in consultation on the farm where she had spent her first five years. While she was a beautiful child, her eyes were wild, nervously scanning her surroundings rather than making contact. Her hair, like her, flew in all directions at once. Her mother, divorced for some years, was increasingly worried about her daughter's odd behavior. In kindergarten Nan stayed on the periphery, playing alone. At home, her bedroom had become a fortress against her anxiety, guarded by toy horses organized in rows according to size and color. Anyone daring to move one risked a furious attack from their trainer. If her arrangement was scattered by a sibling or cleaning efforts, Nan was filled with panic, screaming inconsolably until the horses were returned to their original places. There was no room for error. Her bookshelf was an equestrian collection containing myriad volumes carefully arranged by height and width. On her bed rested a dozen more Percherons, Morgans and Palominos, lying symmetrically, tail to nose, where Nan slept. "Do you want to see my horses?" she asked. I nodded silently and for the next half hour Nan methodically introduced me, by name, to each of her charges on the floor, in the books, on the bed. She insisted that I repeat each name just as she pronounced it. Hard enough for me to experience, this unilateral, compulsive behavior would have totally estranged a five-year-old peer. Nan's passion for order would have discouraged the most ardent lover of horses. It held Nan together, held off mankind.

Obsessive-compulsive behaviors are classified as a form of anxiety. Nan's was nameless panic; Ephraim's was worse. Asked to interview this sixteen-year-old youth for a teaching seminar, I left the classroom to greet him, as was my wont. Standing stiffly erect, tall and thin with bright red hair, he silently refused my outstretched hand. He entered the room but would not sit down, preferring to place himself at a distance from me and the other physicians in the room. He answered my questions in a monotone. "I notice you stand up. Is there any special reason for that?" "Seeping, cosmic poison, germs that cause bad diseases," he answered. "I can't touch them or I'll become very ill." He alluded to threatening voices he heard night and day, their malevolent intent being to bring the world to an end.

We spoke together of the Judgment Day; in time, this topic brought us to the Columbine shootings. "I guess," Ephraim started, "it wasn't such a big deal. It was just political. The guys that died deserved to—rich and spoiled. The papers made too much of it." Ephraim's compulsions and obsessions had lost their struggle with what lay beneath; his was a fractured mind that could, in the right circumstances, become dangerous. His concerns exceeded anxiety; they represented what Bleuler called *Dementia Praecox* or early-onset schizophrenia. His rituals and fears were useless sandbags, failing efforts to stem the rising floodwaters of madness.

Joseph (he insisted on the full name) was a curios mix of humor and pathos. At fourteen he appeared in my office as a slender, odd-mannered youth with an overhanging shock of black hair, dark eyes, a high-pitched, feminine voice with the effeminate gestures to go with it. This likable boy would not enter my office, or remain there, without the presence of his attractive, attentive, divorced mother as his audience and security deposit. The problem, Joseph forthrightly explained, was that certain unmentionable thoughts filled his head to the bursting point. These thoughts had now led him to seriously contemplate suicide. As he recounted this worrisome tale, his mother nodded and smiled, free of any noticeable concern.

With modest encouragement from his mother and me, Joseph filled in the lethal blanks. For some years now he had imagined having sexual intercourse with his mother. He also daydreamed of murdering her with a kitchen knife. These two fantasies had become insistent, obsessional thoughts that felt close to action. Recently, these two themes had been joined by suicidal obsessions that included hanging, jumping, overdosing or slitting his throat with the same knife he imagined using to end his mother's life. Such undisguised imaginings of incest and matricide are frightening to me. They represent primitive impulses close to the act imagined and tell me that the ego is held together by little glue, protected by few filters, and blessed with no malleability—that adaptive mechanisms are impoverished almost to the point of psychotic fragmentation. As I spelled out my serious and relatively urgent concerns for the safety of both mother and son, the mother continued smiling fondly at her son, and pleasantly at me. I took note of the wedding band on Joseph's left hand. He told me that he had never been asked about it before, was not teased about it, and liked the feel of it. He would not consider setting it aside. Mother listened, smiled and nodded in apparent agreement.

This was the Devil's marriage. A misfit son and his single, adoring mother were linked into what in previous times was called a *folie à deux*, madness in a duet. Mother had a permanent partner, a generation younger than she, who gallantly lusted after her, while son had companionship and free access to erotic and violent dreams that, though at time uncomfortable, were a source of entertainment and pride. My posture was one of a humorous wet blanket: I urged mother to approve my recommendations for anti-psychotic medication, a safety plan, and close contact with Joseph's non-physician psychotherapist. The ring was not up for discussion. Fortunately, the mother had enough distance to accept my alarm. Under medication, Joseph's obsessions diminished and became more available for translation by his therapist into more civilized and comprehensible forms. The need to deal with the mother's role was imperative as well. Slowly, psychic breathing space appeared in this x-rated melodrama as the benefits of boredom became evident to both mother and son.

Of course, there are happy compulsions; sometimes, if you believe, they win ballgames. I love baseball and know of misfortune, having grown up a fan of the luckless Chicago Cubs and later becoming addicted to the Red Sox, cursed until 2004.

What are a few harmless rituals if they get you to the World Series? So my son Sam and I watched the great shortstop, Nomar Garciaparra, from out seats in Section Seventeen at Fenway Park. Nomar is a bundle of oddities: he exits the dugout toddler-style, taking pains to place one foot, then the other, on each step. He doesn't change his cap. He never touches a batting weight. He tugs ardently on both batting gloves between pitches and, displaying what is certainly the most copied compulsion of New England Little Leaguers, he alternately taps the toe of each shoe into the dirt of the batter's box three times before the next pitch, a Bojangles Robinson of sport. I ask myself, should his obsessive-compulsive disorder be treated? And ruin his luck, drop his batting average to the low two hundreds, compromise his on-base percentage, his record output of extra-base hits? This is no disorder; this is the exercise of pure talent, establishing continuity over the season, the years—rhythmic rites and rituals that might someday carry Normar to Cooperstown.

Chapter Nine: Humpty Dumpty

Humpy Dumpty sat on a wall,
Humpy Dumpty had a great fall;
All the king's horses
And all the king's men
Couldn't put Humpty Dumpty
Together again.

– Anonymous

No doubt the author of "Humpty Dumpty" had in mind a child psychiatrist rather than an orthopedic surgeon. Broken bones can truly heal, return to their original strength, whereas fractured minds probably cannot. Psychosis and insanity afflict the young of every age. Well before the clay of mind has taken its shape and hardened, it can crack or shatter. The delusions, hallucinations, paranoia, malignant obsessions, mania, thought disorders and suicidal acts in children were described long after their adult counterparts could be found in textbooks and psychiatric hospitals. In the elderly and the young, society tends to minimize signs of psychological trouble by assuming that the illogical and nonsensical are indigenous to those phases of life and need not be noticed or taken seriously.

To further complicate matters, young children normally think in a mode that closely resembles the signs of madness: their lives are replete with imaginary companions, the monsters of nightmares that endure after waking, visions of terrifying intruders, wolves under the bed. All of these and more are the stuff of fairy tales or childhood classics. The first and intrinsically creative mode of thinking common to the early years of life, the "primary process" mode, is guided by impulse, fantasy, wish and symbol, is timeless and has no rules. All things are possible: desires are granted, thunder threatens, giants live. Much of this drama occurs in and around our body, our first and last home. So to decipher this primitive thinking, elegant in its complexity, one needs to rediscover a vocabulary of body contents, all its orifices, their discharges and their remarkable capacities whereby a proudly displayed floating piece of feces is transformed into a penis, a baby or a bomb. Fantasy is fact, inside is outside, and cannibalism as well as every other variety of cruelty, murder, mayhem and annihilation swirl about. Penises can shoot, vaginas can bite, and feces can obliterate. One laughs and takes it seriously; it is play born of imagination, but it is also conviction and sometimes, at a later age, madness.

With the advent of early school age years, from five to seven, primary process thinking is gradually replaced by the logical, limit-bound, reality-based, gray but reassuring presence of the "secondary process" mode that ultimately prevails and, for most, calcifies into civilized decorum. The emerging mental apparatus is fragile, and the capacity of children to test reality accurately, differentiate vivid fantasy from fact, remains unstable well into later childhood, complicating the task of evaluating disturbance. Under duress there are rapid regressions to earlier cognitive styles, often because of illness or the darkness of bedtime. Parents, of course, are flawed diagnosticians, often overlooking, minimizing or denying the obvious, even serious difficulties in their own offspring. Over the years, one of my saddest experiences has been to encounter a child whose psychotic behaviors were never identified in time to prevent irreversible damage, much like fractures that were never set.

Betsy worried her pre-school teachers. An angelic, plump, red-haired three-year-old, she spent increasing amounts of time curled up, masturbating vigorously in the secure corners of the classroom. She related minimally to peers and spoke about "giant black bugs" hunting for her, stalking her. When she played with others it was as if they did not exist; she was the world in its totality. Betsy was conceived at a low point in her parents' marriage, leaving her mother distraught and distracted after her birth. Betsy's development passed as "odd" until her teachers suggested a referral to me. Betsy did not make contact. In my office her precocious but disorganized speech, a staccato fusillade of jumbled words, served to distance her from others. The themes of her utterances were full of danger and violence. I assumed that she was frightened of me and assured her that she was safe in my presence. Her activities were aimless. She moved listlessly but continuously about the room, unable to find repose either alone or with me. Her green eyes looked expressive but only fleetingly met mine. Betsy resembled a larger version of the Energizer Bunny.

Such children require that one violate their personal space to get their attention, wake them up. Left to their own devices, they spin through the universe like satellites without an orbit. Two is a crowd, and intrusive efforts are required to gain entry. While Betsy was an attractive child, she was hard to like; she wasn't there. Her persistent, driven masturbation appeared to be her sole means of self-soothing. In my office was a soft, cream-colored, usually irresistible, bosom-recalling couch. Many children burrowed there, were swaddled there. I sat on it, hoping to attract her to this refuge, but she lay on the floor next to me, stiffening at my quiet entreaties: "You look tired, you could snooze a little, feels good and warm, peaceful." "Big bugs, big biters, in the garden, thunder, thunder" was her answer. After ten or more sessions of my largely one-sided banter, she began to approach the couch, finally mounting its rumpled, inviting cushions; she let me sit next to her there, curled up silently, and fell asleep. This became her therapy: to sleep peacefully in my presence, routine for infants and toddlers, but previously untried and impossible for Betsy.

Her crude, scribbled, heretofore indecipherable drawings began to display recognizable human features, a jagged face with
eyes. This graphic progress paralleled her gradual, halting capacity to make eye contact with me and gently touch my face
with her fingers as would an infant beginning to notice that
her breast milk is not a neighborhood entitlement but delivered by a person. At four, her fund of social cues was meager;
she stood out amongst her peers as different, though her ability to relate with others had improved and her masturbation
was now confined to home. At times she seemed able to share
the world with others. If scared or angry at school, she now
approached her teacher. But Betsy's basic fault lines would not
change. Her best chance for some sort of productive life lay in
learning how to live around them. There are many niches in
this world, and one of my jobs is to help Betsies find a place
where pride in self and acceptance of limitations might be
possible. Trees survive in all seasons and, even if warped or
stunted, continue to grow. They can thrive in unfriendly soil,
though not all are beautiful and many grow aslant.

Psychosis, disintegration of the self, has been variously described. Winnicott, in his spare, sometimes elliptical fashion,
called it "discontinuity of being," ruptures of psychological integrity in time and space. Anna Freud described varieties of
anxiety, one of which she attributed to "the strength of the in-
stincts." The child, conceived of as a vessel displaying variable
tolerance for pressure from within, can sometimes be overwhelmed, flooded by its own impulses or emotions, and begin
to lose its rivets, come apart. In this process the previously
acquired skill of evaluating reality is lost, though sometimes it
was never secured in the first place. It is distressing to witness
a familiar person displaying grotesquely unfamiliar ways.

Albert, an eight-year-old, Eastern European adoptee, had an early history of sadistic abuse and severe neglect at the hands of his addicted, prostitute mother. The scars of cigarette burns were visible on both arms. Referred for his incorrigible lying and stealing, Albert was a lanky, gangly boy whose body never quite seemed to fit him. He was especially attached to a radio he kept by his bed, needing its sounds in order to fall asleep. Albert reported a dream to me: his radio was flying through the air and suddenly broke into pieces that flew in all directions. I felt that this important dream was about Albert, suggesting that he and his most prized possession were one. He and his radio, the source of his only inner peace, had disintegrated, fallen apart and ceased to exist as they once had. After a heavy snowstorm, Albert was delivered to my office by a taxi, which was to pick him up after our session. He was clearly apprehensive about this arrangement and kept peering out of my third floor window so as not to miss his ride. Toward the end of our time, the taxi pulled in early; then, evidently called elsewhere, it turned and drove away. Albert watched with mounting panic, eyes wide with terror, moaning with both hands to the window, lost to any form of contact or comfort from me. If he could have jumped he would have. It was as if the taxi was his last and only means of reunion with his adoptive mother, and it, like his birth mother, had senselessly and abruptly abandoned him. Like the radio in his dream, Albert broke into pieces before my eyes. One of my former teachers believed that anyone could become psychotic if the fear they dreaded most became, even transiently, a reality in their life. For Albert, abandonment threatened the intactness of the self; to be left was to die.

Roadcuts in the region of the Great Eastern Fault, from which brownstone is quarried, sometimes reveal veins of quartz or basalt that disappear after a brief appearance, only to reappear miles down the road in greater abundance, transformed, at times deformed by heat and pressure into new forms with altered characteristics. Likewise, certain vulnerabilities that are present early in children's lives evolve into pervasive, malignant phenomena at later ages. Betty Lou, seven and in second grade, had just moved north from West Virginia. Her parents sought continuing treatment for their daughter's ceaseless agitation. As a toddler she had been acutely sensitive to sounds such as vacuum cleaners, power tools, showers or passing sirens, reacting with panic, putting her fingers in her ears. This hypersensitivity indicated a low stimulus barrier in that part of the brain that screens out and modulates incoming sensations to prevent flooding and confusion. The central nervous system of such children resembles uninsulated wiring, prone to short circuits and overload. Betty Lou was prone to both.

At seven, when I met her, this slight, ethereal girl with a long dress and long blonde hair could have been cut from an art deco poster had it not been for her pulsating anxiety, evident in her urgent voice and manner. In school she was in constant motion, and when sufficiently frightened, simply bolted out of the classroom, running for home if able to reach the outside door. In my office she was the same, standing up, sitting down, moving from chair to chair, startled by sounds, unable to soothe herself long enough to settle. Relating oddly, invading my personal space, and trying to seat herself frenetically on my lap, she proceeded to tell me of her friends Arthur and Doris who had made her "Queen of Zucchiniland." Arthur was "half cat and half monster," Doris "half alien and half frog." I presumed these bizarre creatures were projections of her twisted self, self-portraits *in extremis*.

Her body image was also distorted, perhaps in part from urinary problems in her first year of life requiring repeated catheterizations. She commented: "Something in my front hinie (the family term for vagina) something in there, it's like what makes me swallow and swallow but you don't know about that. It's something that makes you feel like throwing up when you cough." While Betty Lou could not explain her comments, I became concerned that they might reflect sexual abuse, vaginal penetration and/or fellatio. But repeated and detailed questioning was not productive. Psychosis and sexual abuse can be fused and confused with one another or sometimes coexist. She subsequently described auditory hallucinations involving her name being called in a frightening tone and blurred voices whose words and identities were both obscure and confusing. At night she felt angels laying their hands on her shoulders in a comforting way. But during the day there was little comfort; her scattering, bizarre thoughts made concentration and academic mastery impossible, and her odd mannerisms alienated her peers. Winnicott suggested that describing psychosis as "going out of one's mind" was inaccurate and that madness for the most part involved going into one's mind; Betty Lou lived in hers, but neither that chaotic residence nor the outside world she tried increasingly to avoid brought her safety or repose. Her suspicious father permitted me only two meetings with his daughter.

Sebbie was referred to me for assessment of his anxiety. This pale, seemingly studious nine-year-old, unlike Albert or Betty Lou, gave off an aura of calm as he entered my office with his parents; the atmosphere resembled a college admissions interview more than a clinical emergency. Peering at me uneasily through thick lenses, Sebbie listened silently while his mother described his concerns over the past two years. He was certain that his parents were trying to poison him (to which he nodded in agreement), a conviction, growing stronger, that led to elaborate kitchen rituals around mealtime and refusal of all new foods. Sebbie was also concerned that bizarre creatures, half animal, half human surrounded his home at night, circling in wait for their prey outside his windows. He drew crude likenesses of these Goyaesque beasts while, waxing animated, he recited their names. As all of this was communicated to me, I was silent. Sebbie's mother watched me intently and said, "You look worried. Are you?" I nodded. She continued, "You think this is serious." I nodded again. My consultation was over almost before it began.

There are certain situations which, almost at a glance, are clearly grave. Paranoid delusions are exceedingly rare in young children. They usually are seen in violent males who have been sodomized; this was clearly not the case with Sebbie. Here was a well-established, chronic psychosis, an adult-sized disorder strangely out of place in a child's body. Encountering it was like walking through a well-kept neighborhood and, suddenly, coming upon a home burned inexplicably to the ground. I arranged to hospitalize Sebbie on the day I first met him.

One of the saddest parts of my professional work is to bear witness to the slow but inexorable progression of what the great Swiss psychiatrist Eugen Bleuler called *dementia praecox* or schizophrenia. In its most elemental form this illness begins its sluggish ascent in early to mid-adolescence, quietly eroding away and crowding out healthy parts of the self until there remains an almost two-dimensional silhouette of what was—a gray, dull, fearful and avoidant vessel, emptied of its previous contents. This is "process schizophrenia," a formidable and usually victorious opponent, the cancer of child and adolescent psychiatry. What Bleuler felt was a brain disease turns out to be just that, though in its details still elusive. Fifty percent of children who develop this illness show no signs of disturbance prior to puberty; the other fifty percent exhibit varieties of behavioral problems in their early years. But the end result is a death in life, difficult to mourn since the body is still present but certainly not accounted for.

George, at seventeen, was a strong, handsome, muscular youth with closely cropped hair, the kind of boy one would think athletic and popular, riding the mainstream of adolescence. Accompanied by his mother, he walked slowly and stiffly, moving as if through water, and gazing blankly at no one. Until fourteen he was a reasonable student and a fine left-handed pitcher with an extraordinary fastball, good enough to garner two no-hit games. He had a steady girlfriend and was viewed as a leader by his peers. When he entered high school his grades began to falter along with his concentration, and he gradually moved to the social periphery, finding small talk almost impossible. When his girlfriend began dating a classmate, George, already depressed, became desperate as his world passed away before his eyes. On a Saturday night he hid in the woods near his girlfriend's home, ruminating over his fate and jealously watching as her new boyfriend parked and entered her house. Overtaken by rage, he eyed the boyfriend's car for some minutes before stripping naked and knocking on the door Her parents, stunned and frightened, called the police as George fled into the adjoining woods; there he was apprehended in a state of confusion and hospitalized.

On the newer anti-psychotic medicines George became less agitated and paranoid, less convinced that others thought he was gay. He returned home but was no longer able to attend school, now sleeping late into the day, watching television and playing with his younger siblings as might a St. Bernard, not a robust teenager. At night he would roam his house, unable to sleep and at times frightening his parents by walking into their bedroom and standing quietly at the foot of their bed. There is a certain grayness to the skin and sometimes a mousy smell resembling stale sweat or urine that announce chronicity, the sense that some fixed, immobile process with a life of its own has seeped into the pores of the patient, exercising its power like a kind of psychological curare. So appeared George when

I first met him. He was depressed most of the time and aware of how many life functions he had lost. He wept, wondering if he would ever return to his old self but doubting it. A Catholic, he railed at God for giving up on him and felt increasingly that the Devil had won and was within him. He often mentioned suicide but clung to the narrow, constricted life that remained to him. He knew that I liked him but also knew that there was little I or anyone could do to reverse his fortunes.

As a clinician, in the face of graver conditions I can only feel despair at the disruption of a young life where one should see and feel growth and vigor, not deterioration. But it is usually possible to be helpful in some way, at times significantly helpful, and it is always possible to provide comfort. And for me at least, the various paths of lives, both up and down, are in some way beautiful, part of a Nature that mercilessly burns bare her land only to provide life a second, sometimes better chance with second growth. I am not a sailor, but I know the difference between tacking and running with the wind. Psychotic children and adolescents need permission to tack, moving forward by moving laterally, if at all.

My training in psychiatry, unlike that of the present day, involved a curriculum on the dialects and semantics of Bedlam. One of the axioms of my education was that I should follow severely disturbed and psychotic patients for weeks, months or years so as to be at home with the kaleidoscopic, often indecipherable thinking and bizarre, erratic and frightening behaviors of the insane. For those of us with literary interests, this part of our training exposed us to the awesome creativity of the mind. James Joyce became alarmed when Carl Jung diagnosed his daughter as schizophrenic since, he informed the eminent psychiatrist, he thought in the same fractured manner as she did. Jung's considered response: "You dive, she sinks." Benefits notwithstanding, for mature physicians first entering psychiatry, to become at home with madness in adults takes many years and much support.

How, then, is the child with a mentally ill parent to understand and cope with the horrifying transformations that psychosis carries with it? I am certain that Dr. Jekyll and Mr. Hyde were born of experiencing such transformations, and that to compose the mad scene in *Lucia de Lammermoor*, Donizetti must have had first-hand familiarity with the descent from sanity into psychological hell. But they were hugely gifted adults who could transform madness into art. The psychologist Donald Hebb, in his studies on the nature of fear, opined that it is the partially familiar that inspires terror, violation of the expected that provokes dread. Violation of familiar expectancy is precisely what one observes in speech, thought, voice, habitus and facial expression in the decomposition of sanity into madness. One of the fundamental tasks of development in the early years, an essential survival skill, is to establish the capacity to differentiate reality from fantasy or the imaginary, a process usually accomplished by six or seven. However, if a young child's reality is the surreal, shifting, gothic landscape of parental psychosis, the expected is distorted much like images from the mirrors of a fun house. Amy, a sensitive eight-year-old whose mother suffered from an intermittent psychotic disorder, told me quietly, "It's like a bad dream that comes in the daytime when you're not asleep."

Alex, a six-year-old with freckles, copper hair, and a thin mouth that rarely smiled, suffered from that sort of day-mare. His teacher was concerned about his social aloneness and grim mien. It was January and she felt she knew him no better than when school had begun several months earlier. He never spoke of his family, and her questions were met with shrugs or silence. On my first meeting with Alex, I found him sitting stiffly and alone on the waiting room couch. Posture and muscle tone are reliable informants. In a tired, almost bitter tone of voice, he told me that his mother was shopping and would pick him up when we were done. He was unable to acknowledge his natural anxiety in meeting me but moved almost furtively around the office, clearly wary; his eye contact with me was fleeting. When our meeting ended, the waiting room was still empty; I walked Alex to his mother's car.

Later, I met with his parents, both of Scandinavian origin. His mother suffered from Bipolar Disorder (manic-depressive disease) that had appeared in her adolescence. Like many patients with this condition, she was regularly non-compliant with her medication and exhibited bipolarity's characteristic, seismic mood swings. Paralyzed by depression for days at a time, she struggled to manage her family, often unable to rouse herself from bed. To Alex, at these times, she became a distant, unavailable presence. He assumed a caretaker role to cope. Then, without warning, his mother entered the frenzied world of mania: her engine in overdrive, her foot stuck on the accelerator, she became loud, bizarre, suspicious and very angry, always angry. And she rarely slept. Alex had learned to stay out of harm's way until his mother was hospitalized, an interlude that brought both relief and fear. This cycle often repeated itself.

In my office Alex favored drawing to talking. He drew obsessively, depicting an alien planet inhabited by a robot-looking creature that wore a helmet and armored suit much like a land-based deep-sea diver. Tanks and rockets perpetually blasted an unseen enemy. It became evident that the fantasy world Alex recreated on paper was a replica of the life he experienced with his mother, as well as his adaptation to it. Protected from harm by his mental garb, he chose to be alone, and when his mother went out of her mind he went into his; that is where he lived, since there at least he controlled the rules, the laws, the terms of life. His cautiousness about others, his basic distrust, seemed intrinsic to his perceptions—a psychological lens that was not correctable. This visual warp reflected his efforts to fend off his mother on the one hand, since she herself was not trustworthy, and on the other an incorporation of her own perception of the world.

Once I was called by his teacher about a worrisome incident. Alex was passing through the lunch line when he was jostled by another child and responded with a vicious attack on this boy that in its intensity was frightening to onlookers. Psychotic rage is similar. I hoped this was not an early warning sign of emerging bipolar traits and engaged Alex in conversation about the incident: "I guess the kid just bumped you." When he answered "No, he meant to, he wanted to, so he got it," I responded, "You hurt him." Alex answered, "I hope so." Alex and I communicated well with drawing when words failed him. In time he permitted me to pencil in companions to aid in the battle, allowing him to make modest progress toward accepting comfort from friends in his lonely, extra-terrestrial world. Back on earth he became less withdrawn, able at times to enjoy his peers but unable to relinquish either his sense that danger was lurking nearby or his self-perception as an outsider, living on the periphery of life more as an observer than participant. He was rarely invited to birthday parties, an indication of his social isolation. In childhood, perhaps in later life as well, the ability to make and keep true friends is the single most reliable sign of healthy development. The odds are in favor of whoever can do so. Dale Carnegie may have been hokey but he was no dope.

For many children with seriously disturbed parents the family roles are reversed. Propelled by circumstances into premature responsibilities, they parent their parents. This reversal is only present, I believe, in the human species and speaks to the vulnerabilities created by our prolonged childhoods with their needy dependence. The precocious development of coping skills in young children is often as asset in later life, but resentment is always present and the durability of those skills variable at best, since they are furnishings of a first floor perched precariously upon a partially poured foundation.

Alex was a parental caretaker, and so was Margot, seventeen when she sought my help. Successful as a student and competent beyond her years, she had been free of psychological pain until a point in her life when her mother's partner of many years became ill with cancer. Grieving, despairing and desperate, her mother turned again to narcotics for relief, as she had in Margot's early childhood, and regressed to a state of semi-conscious, child-like helplessness. Nursing her mother during the first years of her own life, Margot had learned by three to dial 911 for an ambulance when her mother, stupefied by drugs, became unresponsive. She became night nurse and EMT. The reemergence of her mother's downward spiral had now evoked in Margot the needs that she had so long denied herself and the fury at her mother's failure to meet them. She reported a recurrent, vivid fantasy to me: her mother, dressed beautifully in a rust-colored suit, stood teetering on the floor, with Margot as a child propping her up from behind. To create what appeared to be a normal moment of life, she ran quickly around to face her mother, already beginning to topple backwards, forcing Margot to return to her old and hated task as a prop *in loco parentis*. This fantasy was no mystery to either Margot or me. It was a visual of what she wished for, a mother who could stand on her own rather than the one she had: a mother who asked much, gave little, and intermittently became a troubled child. Like most children with deeply disturbed parents, Margot lived in perpetual dread of a frightening specter: becoming the very person she most despised. It was difficult to dissuade her from the conviction that she was fated to re-publish, without editing, her mother's book of life.

Development is weighted toward life and health; and others in my field have demonstrated that there are many forks in a child's road that can, if available and taken, lead away from the sort of pot-holed routes Alex and Margot traveled: a move to a stronger community, a re-marriage to a loving step-parent, a devoted teacher in a strong school system, athletic talent or marriage to a strong, supportive spouse, to name only a few. Another, of course, is courage in the patient her or himself. I have come to share with the children whom I treat the realization that bad luck abounds in life but that no one will take better care of their lives than they themselves. And while we may own little, if we are fortunate we own ourselves. If nature intended us to look back, she would have placed our eyes in the back of our heads. Besides bitterness, which like Orpheus always looks backward, the most malignant of illnesses in children of any age is passivity: good life outcomes rarely come to those who only stand and wait. Inertia coupled with the "Greyhound" mentality—leave the driving to us—insures paralysis of will, a far graver condition than the diagnosis of major mental illness in a parent or, for that matter, in one's self.

CHAPTER TEN: BAD APPLES

For the imagination of man's heart is evil from his youth. – Genesis 8:21

Child and Adolescent Psychiatry has been furthered by the efforts of devoted, thoughtful juvenile court judges trying to deal effectively with canny, street-smart, wayward youth. As the psychoanalytic model took America by storm in the early Twentieth Century, there was hope that all the ills of mankind, including juvenile crime, might succumb to its curative powers. For good reason, Hope was the last to leave Pandora's Box, presumably because its blindness led to much evil in its own right. Delinquency and anti-social acts predictably defied the psychoanalytic laws of gravity and continued their crooked, maddening and expensive course. Disorders of conduct are, in fact, the most stable of all childhood disturbances over time. They are fiercely resistant to therapeutic intervention. But psychoanalytic students of the anti-social have at least been able to shed light upon the temperamental, developmental and family origins of these conditions.

The questions raised in working with delinquent, criminal children and youth lead one to the deepest ethical, religious and philosophical issues: the origin and nature of evil, social versus biological causes of crime, free will versus determinism, penal versus social/therapeutic programming, the age of criminal responsibility, and the malleability of human character. Debate over these questions resonates through and around our civic, religious and political institutions, opinions swaying to and fro with the passage of generations, historical events and the force of public outcry. For the clinician who enters this archive, the readings are often taken from St. Augustine's entry: "The innocence of children is the weakness of their limbs." With delinquent children the child psychiatrist must be simultaneously hopeful and pessimistic, being certain to differentiate harmless, transient anti-social acts from true criminal behavior and remembering that some delinquency is a symptom suggesting frustration or need rather than a sign of misshapen character.

A credible interpretation of delinquent acts is that they are thoughts or, especially, emotions converted to action. Hence, such acts are translatable if carefully observed. John, a handsome, blond, blue-eyed eight-year-old was referred by a colleague for assessment of his depression and school failure. This bright, energetic child was appealing but not articulate. As with many children, words came to him with difficulty and feelings were inexpressible. He enjoyed chess and relished defeating me, often accurately predicting the number of moves he would need to bring me to my knees. Shortly after beginning therapy with John, I received an urgent call from his mother. He had been caught stealing in a local drugstore, much to her chagrin. I saw John later that day. He drew an odd picture of two mountain peaks between which perched a nest holding a bird with a wide, gaping beak. The mountains resembled breasts.

In taking a more careful history from John's mother, I discovered that his maternal grandmother had been in the terminal stages of cancer during the mother's pregnancy with John. She died when he was three months old. John's mother became clinically depressed before his birth and into the first six months of his life. John's stealing first appeared just prior to a parental vacation when he was six; it recurred a second time at age seven in similar circumstances when a two-week vacation without John was forthcoming. This pattern of minor theft clearly was kindled by the emotional loss of his mother that

John experienced in infancy: his stealing reflected both a need for her and fury at the prospect of losing her again.

John's drawing portrayed, elegantly, a starving infant longing for a feeding that seemed unavailable. If it wasn't given it must be taken. The stolen objects were his just due, owed him by his negligent mother. "John," I said, "maybe we can figure out this stealing business together." As we both looked at his picture, I continued quietly, "When you were a baby your mom was very sad. Her mom died and she missed her; it was hard for your mom to take care of you so you thought she didn't want you, didn't love you." John listened but remained neutral. "And when she goes on vacation, goes away, those old baby feelings come back; you feel mad and don't want her to go. You need her and feel alone and scared when she is gone. That's when you steal." The light of revelation did not pass over my patient's visage. He heard but reserved judgment. But the pattern disappeared. John's basic character was not anti-social. His crimes signaled the breakthrough of feelings of loss and deprivation. The greater part of his development was sound, overshadowing, for the most part encapsulating, the scar tissue of a flawed beginning. With Danny the scar became a keloid.

Danny, a lanky fifteen-year-old boy, walked stoop-shouldered and had dark circles under his eyes. He rarely smiled. He chain-smoked Camels. His gray clothes matched the pallor of his skin, giving him the older, somehow nautical look of a tired stoker from an O'Neil sea play. Danny had been arrested in the subway after breaking into the coin boxes of several candy machines. During his booking he had mentioned suicide often enough to be sent to my hospital. Wary and taciturn, he shared little that would open his life to me. He was an expert lock-picker and had cleaned out coin boxes for many months to generate cigarette money. Danny's family was poor, large and scattered. A wise teacher with whom I discussed Danny suggested that I ask him to teach me to pick locks. This sound counsel capitalized on the centrality of competence in any developing child or adolescent's life.

Pleased to have me as his student, Danny began to tell me of the depth, quality and longevity of his depression. Through most of his life, back to the earliest years, he'd had visions of his "insides" as an empty, pitch black hole, a hollow urn that carried death and despair. At its bleakest this mood was heralded by voices ominously calling out Danny's name in a threatening tone. It was at these moments that he experienced an almost irresistible urge to steal, the act itself partially relieving the bleak night within, turning black into battleship gray. Since theft was the cure, Danny had neither wish nor capacity to give it up and went on to bigger, better and more hazardous self-help. His habit had a life of its own and was a source of pride, not pain, as I learned from a master thief whose trade improved at the owner's peril.

Though Bonnie was as committed to crime as Clyde, until relatively recent times girls and women were in the criminal minority. The anti-social power of woman lay more often in promiscuity, pregnancy, shoplifting and the occasional, Medea-like act of passion. With many shifts in society, family life and equalization, sometimes fusion, of sex roles, more females entered the previously male-dominated, anti-social world. Greta, born in Germany during World War II, was a strikingly beautiful, tall, blonde adolescent who moved and spoke like a young Marlene Dietrich, scornful, seductive, hardened. Her father had served as an officer in the SS, absent, and almost unknown to his daughter. This association with Nazis and the Holocaust was discomforting to me, stirring up my anxiety in her presence. Sexually precocious, Greta entered a torrid relationship at sixteen with a young Rabbi, a chapter in her life she committed to her diary that she left "forgetfully" in reading range upon the family kitchen table. What little remained of a tie to her father abruptly and violently ended. He arranged to send his daughter to America where more distant family members lived.

With family connections but no roots, Greta launched on a career of serious and dangerous acts including major theft, armed robbery and, finally, felony murder. In the company of a male companion, late at night, she attempted to rob a taxi driver at gunpoint. He resisted and Greta, urged on by her partner, shot him in the head. The death was ugly, the crime sufficiently clumsy that Greta was quickly apprehended. Defiant rather than remorseful, she seemed incapable of empathizing with the family of her victim or acknowledging the gravity of her crime. I saw her prior to sentencing. Entering my office she spied a Calla Lily, its green fronds wilting from lack of water. "I hope," she commented bitterly, "you care for people better than you care for plants." I guessed that her attention to the quality of parenting had been learned early and well. She shared little with me. Greta's lust for destruction ran deep, seemingly present since her beginnings.

Certain patients elicit fears in the examining clinician. One learns to take such visceral reactions seriously since they usually signal impulses that lie just short of action. Cory, a seventeen-year-old, exceptionally bright but failing high school senior, big as an NFL middle linebacker, wore black and well-worn, high-top work shoes, shorts and a dirty T-shirt. He was unshaven, sporting a buzz cut and chains: an American skinhead whose manner and appearance contrasted sharply with his verbal nimbleness. Silent and surly, he derided his school's concerns about his dangerousness in monosyllables. Cory scared his classmates and his helpless parents with his mutterings of murder, though he assured me that it was "all in fun." Gory drawings of knives dripping blood or guns pointed at victims had been found in his desk, leading to the referral. Of particular concern was my inability to connect with him and thereby effect any sort of restraint. He sympathized with the Columbine assailants whom he viewed as misunderstood outcasts crying out for help, trying to be "heard." Cory was dangerous. At some point this hulking, rageful, morally impoverished youth would snap, releasing into action the impulses just barely contained in his scribblings. I could only warn his school to watch closely and expel quickly with no margin for error—one strike and he'd be out. Cory planned to enlist in the military for a career that would, I supposed, legitimize his murderous impulses.

When I was in training, a young adolescent boy who had killed his mother was admitted to our hospital. Ordinarily he would have been a patient of mine or one of my fellow residents. But his crime was unnerving to us all, many still struggling with emancipation from ties to our own mothers, so a wise clinical director assigned an older, experienced clinician to his care. Years later I was asked to evaluate Gill, fifteen when he shot and killed his mother. A pale, slight, bespectacled youth, he was soft-spoken and deferential. There had been no warning signs preceding the murder, which occurred during the evening of the day his father and older sister left to visit colleges. His mother had checked his homework with concerns about his failing grades just before the killing occurred. Interviews that detailed Gill's early years, family and school life, and mental state, both current and at the time of the crime, did not reveal any prior disturbance or obvious motive for such a grievous act.

Gill himself, almost apologetic, was at a loss to explain the matricide. Anger, much less homicidal fury, was foreign to his experience. "Tell me about your mom," I said. "She was a hard worker, a good mom." "Do you think she pushed you too hard at times?" "Oh no, I needed it to get my work done." "But you must have been very upset to kill your mom." "I guess so, I don't know." To his neighbors and schoolmates he was helpful, shy but not unpopular, quietly blending in. His father, when I spoke with him, was unable to provide clues to Gill's behavior, though he seemed to me remarkably lacking in grief over his wife's death. He was clear that violence and anger were unknown in his family. But my interview with Gill's older brother was theatrical, grim: after introducing himself to me, settling in his chair, he commented, with feeling, "I like guns, too, you know—they are so powerful. Their power makes them special, beautiful." He loved the touch of oiled, blue steel, but the source of this eerie attraction remained, despite many questions, out of reach.

Completing my contacts with Gill and his family, I could not enlighten his attorney regarding motive and future risk. Some weeks later Gill's father phoned me, in tears, to tell me that he could have shared more but was ashamed. In Gill's early years his mother had cruelly and repeatedly beaten her son for no reason his father knew; a passive man, he'd been unable to stop her. He wondered whether Gill might have harbored long-standing grudges that could explain this otherwise puzzling tragedy. He hoped I would understand his reluctance to share this crucial piece of family history. Clearly, it was enormously relevant. Yet myriads of children suffer extreme physical abuse and never kill anyone, much less their mothers. Our present explanatory models are flawed and incomplete in attempting to explain acts that are inexplicable.

Diego's public lawyer, in search of an expert to testify on his client's behalf, assured me that the boy was "nuts, a head case, certifiably crazy—you'll see." In the lock-up, where I talked with sixteen-year-old Diego in a tiny office, the bright red flush of his cheeks, darting shiny blue eyes, and thick, tousled, blond-orange dyed hair lent him an imago somewhere between innocence and evil. All of his limbs, as well as his words, danced together in a state of agitation, never coming to rest. He fiddled with a glass paperweight on the desk between us, a missile waiting to be launched. I was careful to seat myself close to the office door. Diego's presence spilled noisily over into that of everyone he encountered, instantly provoking fear, anger and retreat. His loud, intense, unmodulated voice poured forth a rapid, steady stream of violent invective at his fellow inmates and the prison staff.

Diego's crime involved the sadistic murder of the grandmother with whom he was living. Prior to killing her, he had stolen silver, jewelry, cash and electronics, hoping to raise enough money to drive cross-country and rejoin his twenty-year-old girlfriend, who had parted with him in anger some days earlier. The theft of these items occurred while his grandmother was out shopping. She returned sooner than Diego expected, startling him and complicating his plans. Enraged by this turn of events, he waited at the top of the stairs, and as she opened the front door he emptied the clip of an assault weapon, some fifteen or more shots raking every part of her body. Taking her car, careening at top speeds, he headed west. He was stopped not far from the murder scene for reckless driving and, the murder weapon at his side, within hours was charged with his grandmother's murder, which he readily admitted.

Diego had been born into chaos. His mother, a drug abuser, left her husband and children without notice when Diego was three. His father, unable to care for his three children, placed them in foster care. In a series of foster homes over the next six years, Diego experienced repeated and severe sexual molestation, sodomy in particular, as well as brutal physical assaults from foster siblings. Already practiced in theft, fire-setting, and cruel treatment of animals, childhood markers of trouble to come, he now became a skilled, wily, sexual predator preying upon younger occupants of his foster homes. Pre-pubertal boys who have been sodomized inflict, with particular pleasure, the cruelest acts upon others. Diego was no exception. He described, with obvious relish, his hateful, remorseless, childhood exploits. As for his grandmother, the meddlesome "bitch," she was too strict, too tight with money and, on the day of her death, a bothersome glitch in his plans. He had planned to kill her, just not at this time, but once started, he felt gleeful pleasure in watching his last blood relative, one who genuinely cared for him, writhe in agony, bleed profusely, and expire at his feet without a sound.

Diego met all the criteria of sanity in the formal psychiatric sense. His attorney was furious, certain that I, at least, was "off my rocker." What I believed and told him was that his client enjoyed killing and that this pleasure was uninhibited by any signs of conscience or remorse, that he had virtually no control over his impulses. What he felt was what he did. Diego was, therefore, extremely dangerous to society and would remain so indefinitely. Since his prognosis was so poor, and since medication and other therapies were of such minimal use, I recommended that Diego remain in a locked facility for the foreseeable future. Medication and supportive counseling would comfort him but alter neither his character nor his dangerousness. While one could credibly account for Diego's profile with a combination of biological and familial data, to me he was evil, a guiltless, sadistic killer who enjoyed taking lives, for whom the pleasure of destruction would always remain an inexorable force. Those who believe, as I do, that crimes of this nature and magnitude rely upon a free-standing capacity for evil may conclude that Eve's apple, that bad apple, did not fall far from its tree.

It is, however, important to distinguish between basic evil and temporary error. Many years ago I served on the Admissions Screening Committee at Tufts University School of Medicine where I worked and taught for twenty years. The involvement of psychiatrists in the admission process was based on the presumption that our knowledge and skills would serve to identify and eliminate poor risks from the student body. One candidate for admission, a young man in his early twenties, deeply committed to a career in medicine, made a good contact with me and shared much that was personal. Like most of us, he was eager to talk if there was an ear to truly listen. His father had died when he was sixteen, a sorrow clearly still with him. He and his family had struggled to make ends meet and he had made it through college on scholarships and jobs on the side. Then, he said, he wanted to tell me something that might jeopardize his career. Would I inform the rest of the Committee or would this information remain confidential? I told him that I would have to use my discretion and reminded him that my mission was to serve the School, not him. Red-faced, squirming, he told me that he had stolen a motorcycle after his father's death, an expensive Harley-Davidson that he claimed as his own. Our interview ended shortly thereafter. I thought about this young man's life, past and present. I thought about the many candidates who had told me nothing of their misdemeanors, who had been alert to the politics of the process. I liked this man and knew fundamentally that he was not a criminal, that in fact he was of good character and long on determination. His theft seemed to me an act of restitution in the aftermath of his father's death. I recommended him for admission.

Fifteen years later, when we lived in the same community, he spied me on the street. He told me, with obvious pride, that he had become a surgeon and was now practicing locally. He thanked me for my confidence in him. I was not surprised, but I was deeply moved to think that his life had gone forward so well for him and for those whom he served and would continue to serve, making their care his life's work. It was a little thing; it was a big thing. A shot at life is a big thing.

Chapter Eleven: Family Matters

Happy families are all alike; every unhappy family is unhappy in its own way. –Leo Tolstoy

The family system is not intrinsically benign. Dysfunction is, given the nature of man, inherent in its structure. It is endowed with enormous power to facilitate but also stunt and sometimes destroy the forward trajectory of a child's life. In the belly of the family is a child psychiatrist's diagnostic and therapeutic overlook. From this vantage point the possibilities for change are sized up and, when possible, put in motion. Working knowledge and artful, nuanced skill in shifting the frozen gears of family systems are major levers for freeing up a child's developmental energies. But layman or professional, we are all limited by the imprints and echoes of our own families. A colleague of mine in Boston, a highly respected family therapist, decided to try repairing the damage in his family of origin by gathering them together in Manhattan where they lived. On the Massachusetts Turnpike, en route to this event, he fell asleep at the wheel, narrowly avoiding a serious accident. Assuming that Fate was warning him, he returned home to try again. On his second attempt a similar scenario repeated itself. Wisely ending this venture, launched in the spirit of "physician heal thyself," my colleague, somewhat sheepishly, acknowledged that in facing his family he was flooded with emotions too powerful to be contained. How many of us, I have often wondered, could express with candor to our parents and siblings the accumulated grievances, past and present, of our family life?

Family has its darker sides. To Alexander Pope it was a "commonwealth of malignants"; to Strindberg it was the place "where innocent children are tortured...where wills are broken by parental tyranny, and self-respect smothered by crowded, jostling egos." While we know of and often idealize the family's power for the good, we sometimes ignore its destructive influences. The truth of family lies, perhaps, somewhere in between. One of modern psychiatry's great contributions to understanding human behavior in general, and the development of health and illness in children in particular, is the creation of a vast amount of observational data on family systems and the laws that govern them. The original models of family as an interactive system were borrowed from Werner von Braun's investigations into missiles and rockets, appropriately identifying family with a category of dangerous explosives. Studies of families have led to family therapies, interventions treating the entire system as patient; other research has contributed to an increasingly refined knowledge of the specific contributions of family processes to the shaping and emergence of psychiatric disorders in childhood and adolescence. In the last forty years many rich and testable hypotheses have been generated, some directly applicable to the practice of child psychiatry.

Adelaide Johnson and Stanley Szurek studied the families of children who exhibited anti-social behaviors, interested in understanding the parental sanctioning of delinquency. Over several years of observation they formulated their now classical hypothesis that deficiencies of conscience in one or both parents, what they called *superego lacunae* (like the holes in Swiss cheese), lead to ambiguous, "mixed" communications to the child that are heard as invitations to carry out the very acts simultaneously discouraged or prohibited. Somehow, the valence of permission to engage in anti-social behavior mutes or extinguishes the prohibition against it.

An example: the father of a nubile, adolescent daughter, struggling with his own sexual feelings and aroused by her pubescence, constantly criticizes her boyfriends and is suspicious that she is sexually involved with them. His distress is articulated with comments to his daughter such as "you little slut," or "next thing you know you'll be home with a baby." The overt content of these messages is "be careful, control yourself," but the powerful, covert content is a call to action: "Go and get pregnant." In a diagnostic evaluation of my own, I interviewed a six-year-old fire-setter with his mother. She assured me that she and his father were strict and clear with their son about the danger of matches. In the midst of that assurance she pulled out a cigarette. As if on command, her son wordlessly plucked the pack of matches from her hand and, executing an obviously well-practiced ritual, struck and lit one as his mother leaned over to accept his adeptly delivered assistance.

It happens in the best of families. On a Sunday afternoon I was called by a professor's wife, in tears, desperate to stop her husband from beating their twelve-year-old, honors student son. As we spoke she held the phone out so that his screams could be heard from the basement where his father had taken him to receive his punishment. On discovering that fifty dollars was missing from his dresser, her husband had grabbed the boy, shaken him and accused him of the theft. A forced confession provoked the paternal rage that I was overhearing. Mother refused, in shame, to call the police. I insisted that she put her husband on the phone. A furious voice told me to mind my own business. I identified myself as a colleague and told him that unless he stopped the assault immediately, I would be obliged to call the police. A long silence ensued, then a grudging "okay." I asked that he, his wife and son come to my office. He waffled, I insisted.

Their son, Rob, was a slender, athletic boy, tall and handsome, dressed casually in a uniform of the well-to-do. His face was flushed, bruises evident on his cheeks. His father, whom I greeted with a firm, respectful handshake that he returned, was a striking man, out of central casting for English gentry. Rob's mother, pale and tearful, was a lady in dress and manner. I met alone with Rob who, despite my assurance of privacy, took the Fifth Amendment. I invited his parents in. "Fill me in," I began. The father wasted no time: "The little bastard stole a wad from me, right under my nose. What," he asked, "would you do if it was your son?" "I hope not thrash him. In my family that's off limits and it ought to be in yours. Where," I asked, "do you keep your money?" As the narrative unfolded it became clear that the top of the father's dresser was the family ATM. His change and his folding money lay there, uncounted and unaccounted for except on rare occasions. Both mother and son availed themselves of these funds on a regular basis without acknowledgment on their part or protest on the father's. Occasional paternal rampages, such as had just transpired, were unconvincing since his banking practices never changed for more than a day or so. Honesty and integrity, I was assured, were shared family values. Rob was stuck; so was I. In this silent, persistent scenario, who was the patient? Father, mother, son or family unit? My mandatory reporting to the Department of Social Services affected only a temporary lull in the pattern of family cash flow.

The clinical accuracy and predictive power of the Johnson/Szurek hypothesis is quite remarkable. When I see patterns of family communication such as just described, I know immediately that delinquent acts by the children involved (theft, vandalism, sexual promiscuity, firesetting, etc.) are enmeshed in a family process whose faults are both patently obvious to observers and remarkably obscure, inaccessible to family members, even when identified. The power of unconscious impulses shared and amplified in a family system is such that efforts on my part to illuminate, not to mention modify the system, will fall on deaf ears. In fact, there is little or nothing I can do to alter delinquent behavior despite a bird's-eye view of its causal agents. I hold the lock, know the combination, but cannot open the shackle. The disorders of conduct bred by dysfunctioning families seem immune to any known psychotherapies. They are a stable historical presence over many generations. Eve, after all, was not given the apple. She took it. Man's "first disobedience" was not his last.

Salvatore Minuchin and his colleagues came at the family system from another direction. Their observations suggested that there was a continuum of family interactive styles that, if known, would predict the diagnostic profiles of the children in any family. The "Disengaged" family system they characterized by the isolation of its members from one another, like right and left hands quite unaware of each other's plans. Syndromes of action and impulse, externalizing disorders seem to be associated with Disengagement: conduct disorders, anti-social personalities, and alcohol or substance abuse In one such family that I saw in a teaching conference, husband and wife rarely spoke; there were no common mealtimes, and neither was familiar with the children's teachers. Sean, the oldest son, nineteen, drug-addicted and unemployed, had not been seen for some weeks by his family. He returned silently to the family home and hung himself in the basement while life above went on as usual. No one in the family was aware that Sean was in town, had come home, or was suicidally depressed.

In contrast, the "Enmeshed" family style described by Minuchin exhibits poor interpersonal boundaries, little differentiation of one member from another, minimal autonomy in the children, and little or no privacy. *My business is your business. My phone call, conversation, mail and sometimes thoughts are yours.* Here one finds internalizing disorders such as depression, anxiety, psychosis and psychosomatic syndromes. David, eighteen, returned home after only a month of his first year in college, having been described as "anxious" by the college counseling center. His mother called for an emergency appointment. David was tall, skinny, homely and paranoid. Acutely schizophrenic, he was given anti-psychotic medication in my office some hours before he was hospitalized. The next day his mother called to ask that I meet with her and her husband immediately. The night of David's admission to inpatient care, she noticed that his father had suddenly developed the precise throat-clearing mannerism that David displayed. Based upon this single piece of data, she concluded that her husband was, quite literally, turning into David, becoming psychotic, and began giving him the remaining doses of the medication I'd prescribed for her son. Psychologically fused with David, unable to tolerate his absence, she instantly transformed her husband into her missing child to re-establish equilibrium in the family system. In this family, even with a scorecard, one couldn't know the players.

I have found Minuchin's ideas useful but over-simplified. There are few families within which enmeshment or disengagement exist in anything approaching pure culture. Most families display some elements of both.

The ancient warning that "those whom the Gods would destroy they first make mad" needs revision in light of family systems theory: those whom families must keep, to maintain the integrity of the parental relationship, they make mad or, if already impaired, resist repairing. The ill wind of a disturbed or otherwise chronically ill child often blows one or both parents good. They can unite in a common, never-ending project, or join forces against an outside enemy, thus distracting them from the bankruptcy of their marriage and the dissolution of the family. To child psychiatrists this counter-intuitive dynamic is commonplace. To parents who may become aware that helpfulness to the ill child carries with it the high stakes of marital dissolution, the insight is unwelcome and alarming. Its cold, fluorescent, truthful glow often lies buried beneath but at the center of the noise and tumult of a family's life.

Pat was, at twelve, the oldest of three children in an apparently well-knit family. Father, an attorney, appeared invested in his son's life but never quite followed through with the steps to help Pat in his failing academic pursuits and social estrangement. Pat was his mother's full-time project. Chauffeur, tutor and social secretary, she nonetheless complained bitterly about his endless needs and lack of progress. Seen together, his parents behaved much like Penelope in Homer's Odyssey, unraveling during the night what she had woven earlier that day, moving nowhere with deliberation. From confusion and uncertainty about how much to supervise Pat's errant studies or what his punishments should be for incomplete work, they moved with me to a concrete plan of action by our session's end. When we reconvened two weeks later it was as if no plan had been formulated. They took each other and me to task for not knowing how to deal with Pat's school problems and appeared as confused as before. The confusion of the parents was not relieved by my "but don't you remember?"

In their interactions with one another, as we sorted through the confusion, the father waxed increasingly angry at his wife, scornful of her efforts, which he belittled. Shortly reduced to tears, she implored her mate to guide her, tell her what to do. I saw that the father was fed up with his spouse; his dislike was a palpable presence. Sensing his rancor, the mother wept, sank down in her chair, turned paler. After several cycles of this pattern, I wondered out loud with Pat's parents if they might be struggling with issues of their own, unrelated to Pat but within which he might be caught. My gentle, tentative query was met with blank looks. They accepted my referral to a marital counselor but after two sessions found her schedule, her fees and, most of all, her questions "unrelated to Pat's difficulties." While they agreed that every couple could benefit from someone like her, they spoke as one in saying that their priorities were with Pat. Their son, however, keeper of the family glue, expensive glue, deteriorated. He was as unreachable to me as were his parents. All began to wonder out loud whether this "therapy stuff" was worth the trouble but, with one foot out the door, continued. I knew that my hands were tied, as were Pat's, and tactfully ended my fruitless efforts.

At a more primitive level, Arnie was the first of my patients to instruct me in the (unconscious) parental motivation to drive a child crazy. A big, burly, unshaven eighteen-year-old with the look of a homeless person and a scathing sense of humor, he had been hospitalized for many months with paralyzing obsessional ruminations and accompanying despair. We liked one another, and Arnie knew that I appreciated his wry, daily commentary on the state of his ward, my sartorial habits, and his family. In our weekly meetings he would remark, "My father is trying to kill me," or "My goddamn mother makes me nuts, certified nuts." Having made and heard similar comments over the years, I initially discounted Arnie's gripes as relatively standard fare. Then I met his parents and listened more astutely to my patient's frightening but credible allegations.

Arnie was the last of four children; his older siblings had all left home and appeared to be reasonably successful. His father, a small, intense, dapper man, a Mutt to Arnie's Jeff, wore a chronic scowl. In Arnie's presence he praised his son's unsuccessful efforts at autonomy, immediately undoing his support with comments like "Arnie can't fight his way out of a paper bag," or "Anyone dressed like this slob is going nowhere fast," and "How did I grow a son like this? I don't think he's mine." All of this was directed to me but within easy earshot of his son. For me it was painful and infuriating. Arnie's mother, doughty and bland, stood nodding in compliance with her dominating spouse. Arnie had told me previously, "She's useless." At this moment I had to agree.

In a session with me shortly after this meeting, Arnie described a weekend at home with his parents. On Sunday his father had parked across the street, a heavily trafficked highway, from the restaurant where they were dining. His parents crossed quickly, a feat Arnie could never match since he took two steps back for every one forward as he traveled in his obsessional manner through this world. At the moment he garnered enough forward momentum to join them, his father began a series of commands: "Quick, now...no, wait...step on it...Jesus Christ what is the matter with you?...look out, you idiot, don't you see that car...you are a hopeless, hopeless fuck-up...you'll never make it in life." So rapid, so confusing and so destructive was this coaching that Arnie, enraged and terrified, walked home, leaving his parents to dine alone.

This was vintage according to Arnie. His father's public, humiliating diatribe that led to confusion, fury, and ultimately paralysis and despair was a pattern that he had incorporated wholesale into the few remaining fragments of a vestigial self and a vertiginous view of the world that left life perpetually spinning out of control. Later that year Arnie phoned me on a Sunday afternoon. I could not identify the screaming voice: "I can't take it anymore. Please, Dr. Robson, you've got to help me, you've got to stop them...(prolonged, rageful, desperate screaming, closest, perhaps, to that of a bull elephant)...I can't take it anymore." Arnie was in the midst of another interaction with his family. In fact, he could not take any more and was transferred the next day to the State Hospital where he remained, lifeless, thereafter. I thought of it as soul murder. According to Dr. Harold Searles, a gifted student of the chronically mentally ill, a primary motive for creating insanity in a loved one is to ensure his or her constant presence and prevent the loved one from ever evolving a life or a self, so that the architect of madness might himself remain whole, and never alone.

Families, more than their individual members, are idealized; it seems somehow easier to acknowledge and accept the flaws of a mother, father, brother, sister or grandparent than to find fault with the family itself. Denial seems to thrive better in the plural than the singular. R.D. Laing, a briefly famous British psychiatrist, took the unpopular position in his studies of chronic schizophrenia that the family system is inherently destructive to the development of its individual members, that it can maintain coherence and survive only at the expense of those members, particularly the children. In part, Laing is right. But Winston Churchill, his fellow countryman, whose own family was a disaster, commented that "It has been said that Democracy is the worst form of government except all those other forms that have been tried from time to time." Most would agree, especially on rainy days, that the same can be said of family.

I believe that child and adolescent psychiatrists are biased toward focusing on the omissions or commissions of the families we deal with and help. There is a nameless law that trouble is noisier and more visible than the sound of what is working properly. This was true even in medical school where illness and bizarre symptoms fascinated us while public health and prevention put us to sleep. But nothing is more rewarding than seeing a patient regain equilibrium.

Robin's mother and step-father wept when they shared with me the events of their five-year-old daughter's short life. When she was three her father was killed in Vietnam. One year later she developed the symptoms of ulcerative colitis: multiple bloody stools, painful cramping and trips to the emergency room by ambulance. The hospital was not a refuge either: Robin suffered the indignities of colonoscopies, intravenous treatments and the jabbing and poking her condition required. Not surprisingly, Robin developed states of panic and despair that had become another chronic illness by the time I saw her at five. She had become fearful of the world, had withdrawn from friends, and had lost confidence in herself. She was miserable.

Robin was a beautiful child. What struck me most was her wide, inviting smile that said, "I'm ready." It was so at odds with what her parents had described to me. Like many children who are exposed to illness early in life, she was verbally precocious. "My dad," she said, "told me you would help me, Dr. Robson. I'm a mess of trouble but I don't want to be." And she wept.

Robin received a new pink bicycle for her birthday. She refused to ride it, despite the training wheels in place and despite her parents' patient reassurance. There are central metaphors in many therapies, and the bicycle became a shared symbol for Robin, her parents and me. With my own children someone (long forgotten) had taught me to use a rolled up beach towel around a child's waist to produce stability from behind as the child gains confidence in riding alone, first with training wheels, then alone. Daily throughout her fifth year, mother in the morning, father when he returned from work in the evening, held Robin upright as she wobbled, beach-toweled, towards competence. Her parents needed only the slightest shove from me to get their wheels turning. There was protest and dread, but Robin cut a deal with me — if she really wanted to "clean up the mess" she'd have to do the sweeping. I gave her a wet mop to put in the garage next to her bike to remind her of our contract.

At summer's end she gleefully rode on her own just before her sixth birthday. Pride goeth before many falls off a two-wheeler. But by seven she was an ardent cyclist without training wheels. She and her step-father made excursions together. Robin's success was a family venture and a family gain that set in motion the latent assets Robin owned. The beach towel, in the right hands, dried her tears and set her on a steady course of her own. At age twelve, while still on cortico-steroids, Robin entered adolescence passing her peers on the curves. Her joy was infectious to her family and to me. While her colitis stabilized, she continued to suffer flare-ups of painful, bloody diarrhea, but the panic diminished. She surrounded herself with friends and school went well. Robin imagined a career in pediatrics. Her family's staunch muscle held this child and let her go in a way that was perfectly choreographed. Like Nureyev holding Fonteyn.

CHAPTER TWELVE: HOUSES DIVIDED

When I can no longer bear to think of the victims of broken homes, I begin to think of the victims of intact ones.

– Peter De Vries

A substantial amount of my practice involves conducting custody studies in contested divorces when the parents are in total disagreement regarding a plan of care for their minor children. The vast majority of divorces require no intervention, since parents generally resolve their post-divorce lives amicably. Because I am an experienced child psychiatrist, I attract referrals in the most difficult and acrimonious cases. While many "intact" families are rife with endless conflict, in divorce one may see, fully exposed, particular configurations of family life that can drastically reshape children's futures. Just as with Arnie, a parent can destroy his child, and in cases of "parental alienation," one parent can effectively destroy the other, a profound loss for any child. Alienation can be motivated by both conscious and unconscious impulses or needs including revenge, dread of losing one's children, or the wish to be the only one. Regardless of motive, if alienation is successful, the end result is elimination of one parent from a child's world. I consider this situation an emergency since there comes, in all of these cases, a point of no return where the process of alienation cannot be arrested, much less reversed.

The Jorgensens had never been a happy family through the fifteen years of their marriage. When Marie filed for divorce, the three Jorgensen daughters, Karen seventeen, Crista fourteen and Alma ten, were not surprised. They had borne constant witness to their parents' vitriolic, sometimes physical strife. The girls were relieved. Their father Eric, however, was taken by surprise when papers were served on him. He responded with seething anger at Marie, bitter hurt that hardened into payback, a guiding mantra he had warned her of many times: "Lose me, lose your girls." Spurned by a wife he did not love, his rejection-sensitivity reorganized his life around retribution for being asked to leave a party he no longer wanted to attend. Like an elephant, Eric never forgot. He made certain that his audience, Karen, Crista and Alma, didn't either.

The initial Massachusetts court orders in the Jorgensen divorce recognized Marie's competence as a full-time, stay-at-home mother. The girls lived with her in the family home on Boston's North Shore, residing with Eric on alternating weekends. By the time I became involved, directed to complete the custody study, Karen had become totally estranged from her mother. She refused to see or communicate with Marie and now lived with her younger sisters in the same home but with Eric as primary parent. Karen would not meet with me, the two remaining sisters doing so under protest. My office could have been Salem during the witch-hunts. Alternately, Crista and Alma alleged: "Mom is nuts. You don't believe us but she is truly cracked; she hates us, too." Then, in the precise words used by Eric, like a grim Greek chorus, they continued: "She hates dad, too; she had no business breaking up our family. She's a busybody, she meddles in our lives. You better listen to us, no one else does; we don't want to see her anymore, just once in a while when we want to, that's enough." Crista by now was on the verge of relinquishing her ties to her mother while Alma was still ambivalent.

Marie had given me several home videos from summers on Nantucket. I reviewed them with care. It was obvious that the children were loved by her and loved her; there was no mistaking the delight all three girls displayed, over the years, in their mother's company. But Eric's relentless vendetta against her and her own helpless passivity combined to reduce Marie's power to virtually nothing in the battle for the hearts and minds of her girls. I completed my study and issued a report that recommended drastic action: Marie was to resume primary custody and Eric's time was reduced to allow some neutralization to occur. If there was evidence of continuing devaluation of Marie on his part, the girls would see him only with a neutral supervisor present to monitor his communication and, if necessary, terminate the visit. Technical matters delayed the implementation of my report's recommendations. By the time that occurred, both Crista and Alma had joined their sister in excluding Marie from their lives. A tearful Marie saw me repeatedly, asking for guidance, but no strategies were effective. When I met with her for the last time, she had become resigned to having no contact with the girls but held out the hope that as adults they might "come around." I did not share her expectations for the future. Antidotes to Eric's distorted, egocentric toxins were not on the market. Saddest to me was the loss of a good mother to these children. She had not been claimed by death; she loved them deeply but was dead to them in life.

The great majority of children of divorce wish, most of all, for parental reunion, a longing that rarely reflects an accurate memory of the familial misery that preceded a separation or divorce. Liam wished for no such resolution to his parents' divorce. When we first met he owned an "old soul" stowed in a short frame topped by an unruly shock of black hair. The rigidity of his alignment with his mother concerned me, since my mission was to preserve access for him to the best that both parents could muster. Then I met his father. "He's nuts. He says he loves me but he doesn't. He's mean, wanna hear?" I shrugged. Liam went on to describe a frightening scene in the parking lot where his father picked him up on the weekends, few and far between, that he spent with his son.

Liam's dad had an explosive, mercurial temper that was a prime mover in his mother's decision to dissolve the marriage of fifteen years. Over those years he had terrorized his wife and three sons with destruction of walls, smashing of windows and, on occasion, physical violence that led to police involvement. On the Saturday morning in question, his mother and father squabbled through open car windows over the time of the boy's return on Sunday. In a rage, the father began a car chase around the parking lot, colliding with his wife's rear bumper when he could. Court orders temporarily suspended father-son contact.

An intelligent but brittle man, Liam's father towered above me. He was very tall though not imposing, his volcanic nature well wrapped. While he claimed to love all of his children, he was oblivious to the impact on Liam of his wrathful ways, broken promises and erratic appearances. Bitter about the divorce, righteous in his denials, he spent his time with me berating his wife; a listener might have concluded he was childless. In some way his tie to Liam was deficient and his parental heart in the wrong place. He was also dangerous. I came away from this contact wondering if Liam's exit wishes might not be well-founded.

At our next session Liam seemed frightened; he burst into tears and wept wordlessly for a time. "He will get me, Dr. Robson, he will; he won't stop until I move in with him. I hate him. He never cared when he was around and he doesn't now." His voice rose to a scream: "I hate him, I never want to see him again, I want to cut him out of my life...cut, cut, cut..." Here he lost control, picking up a chair and trying to throw it across the room, his face contorted with anguish. I restrained him and he calmed in time. He knew my office rules: no one gets hurt, nothing gets broken; but in this instance they failed to contain him. I was watching a down-scaled version of his father, caught inside like a bad, permanently undigested meal. Liam looked at me imploringly: "I hear him all the time, calling my name, yelling my name." "In your head?" I asked. He nodded and began to cry again. "Do you think about dying?" He nodded again and shared with me that he had thought about running into traffic. I decided that he needed hospitalization.

There is no getting away from a parent who terrifies. Though across the world, such a parent remains ensconced within a child. Often that part of one's identity remains latent until later in life when it can erupt quite suddenly when the strain of parenthood begins. The mechanism for such an unfortunate piece of one's psychic anatomy was seen in the Holocaust. The Jewish guards, "Kapos," unconsciously adopted the sadistic ways of their Nazi keepers, at times outdoing them in their torment of fellow Jews in the Camps. Reports after the war expressed disbelief, repugnance and amazement at this seemingly bizarre behavioral display, but unfortunately Nature seems to have invented only one mental mechanism to master terror's assault upon one's being. Its formal title is identification with the aggressor, a rigid, primitive means of adaptation, coping or defense. Children can be selective in deciding whom they love, but they have no control over whom they hate.

Liam profited from his stay in hospital and was started on anti-psychotic medication to help his tenuous equilibrium. His father knew of Liam's distress but did not visit him. A kindlier Fate brought his mother into a new relationship with a gentle man who was genuinely invested in Liam's life and sensitive to his needs. He brought with him an auxiliary therapist in the form of a golden retriever named Jack, whom Liam quickly came to love. Jack slept on Liam's bed and listened in the way only dogs can. I discouraged Liam from any more vitriolic debasement of his father, concerned that it would preclude any possibility of a reconciliation in the years to come. Ties matter, even when frayed. Liam was too young to know what he might need or even want down the road.

The Underground Railway that carried runaway slaves to the North had a major stop in Boston. It was a force to be reckoned with. Reborn in the Twentieth Century, a new model of this clandestine travel transports divorcing parents and their children out of Boston to escape a variety of evils attributed to the parent left behind. The Cohen girls were passengers at the time I became involved in their parents' ugly dispute. Lily was eight, Hannah eleven when their mother, Laura, fled the family home with them. Because federal kidnapping charges were leveled against Laura, the FBI was involved in tracking mother and daughters down in Cuba, their last stop on a labyrinthine journey. The network that supported Laura Cohen, and numerous others like her, is vast and well endowed. Its backers share common beliefs in the corrupt state of our legal system and the excessive powers of government. They were, therefore, sympathetic to Laura's profound concern that her husband Art was involved in serious, ongoing sexual molestation of both of their daughters. These allegations were not substantiated in court. It was in this context that, as a last resort, Laura fled. The escape didn't last long.

Hannah was suspicious of my every move. Short and stocky with black, curly hair, she followed me like radar with her dark eyes. Her lips pursed tightly in a silent, stubborn scowl. Lily was a smaller version of her sister but seemed at ease with herself, more sociable, more trusting. While the details of their experiences were never disclosed to me, I knew that both girls had lived in hiding with confusion and anxiety. In my initial meetings with them I simply let them "hang out" with me, explore the office, play cards, examine my dolls, and eat or drink. I posed virtually no questions to them, hoping to create an atmosphere of safety and neutrality. I knew they were confused about my role as one of the many anonymous players who had assumed bit parts in the drama of their lives during the past year. To be enigmatically benign, ask nothing of them, seemed to me a kindly strategy to avoid their confusing me with whoever and whatever had gone before.

Lily was happy to engage: "You're here to take our mom away from us so we can live with dad. Mom is in jail." Hannah stood behind her sister, whispering, coaching, monitoring her every word. She was the prompter in this libretto. "I know you guys don't know me, but my job is to help figure out with your mom and dad, and the judge, what's going to help you the most now that you're home again." Lily nodded, smiled while Hannah countered "I know what—you're a spy to keep my mom in jail. You don't know what our dad did to us all the time. We hate him and we're never gonna live with him—he hurt us a lot." "Yeah," echoed Hannah in a rote manner that was to recur frequently, "he hurt us all the time." "Well, whatever happened before, you're safe now and part of my job is to be sure that no one hurts you." I invited the girls to play Old Maid. Lily joined me on the floor but Hannah, flustered and torn, held back. I had begun to establish my "straight man" role.

The girls lived with a maternal uncle and aunt outside Boston while around them swirled a myriad of court proceedings. During this time I met with both parents alone to make contact and gather history. Laura, in appearance, was a clone of her daughters. She was a one-woman wire service, providing vast numbers of documents describing her courage in protecting her children from their father's carnal lust. Many hours were spent establishing a chronology of events, the paternal narratives diverging sharply. Art was a large, brusque but kind-hearted man who shunned the public eye and seemed very concerned about his daughters' traumatic journey. In several meetings with Laura and her daughters, their closeness was evident. Hannah, the appointed or self-appointed stool pigeon, made her mother aware of my "sneaky questions" and made certain she knew that "he doesn't think anything happened to us with dad; he doesn't believe us." Having said nothing of this kind, I wondered whose opinion her words reflected. Perhaps her own?

My initial meeting with Art and the girls required much preparatory effort. They had not seen their father for more than a year, though historically he had been involved deeply in their lives. He brought favorite, well-worn toys and a craft project to this session. I had warned Art to avoid defending himself should either or both girls use this contact to renew their allegations of abuse, face to face, with the "perpetrator." Lily was clearly thrilled to see her father, jumping into his arms, delivering a long hug and "I missed you, daddy." As Art then welcomed Hannah, she withdrew to the back of the office and, pointing her forefinger at him, began his prosecution: "You're just trying to fool us again. You hurt us." Lily, as a barely audible chorus, repeated "You did hurt us." Hannah went on: "You want to take us away from mommy. You want to hurt us again, again, again." Lily, holding Art's hand tightly, nodded her assent during this diatribe. Art, heeding my warning, spread a blanket on the floor and began the project he had carried with him. Neither child could resist, and they joined him.

Over several weeks I met with the girls to try and document their heinous allegations that included multiple episodes of sodomy, fellatio and vaginal penetration. There are physical findings that suggest such violence. The examinations I requested on both children were negative. And while neither child could describe the details of a particular date, time, place clothing worn etc., I knew that embellished, melodramatic stories can contain a nidus of documentable truth and was mindful of my primary responsibility for these children's present and future safety.

Hannah again and again accused Art of sodomizing her repeatedly, while Lily looked on. On one occasion Hannah was weaving in new details when, suddenly, Lily said quietly, "We faked it, we faked it all." Hannah, more startled than I, turned to her sister with a shocked, quizzical look. I continued, "I heard you, Lily, but now I'm mixed up; I'm not sure what happened." Lily, again: "We faked it all, all the time we faked it." Now Hannah, unable to contain herself, stared at her sister and queried, "Well, did it happen or didn't it? I'm mixed up now too." Lily and I were silent; Hannah looked confused and repeated her questions to Lily twice more. Then, turning to me she uttered, "It did happen. I know it and you don't believe it." "Well," I responded, "I'm confused. So is Lily and so are you." This dramatic turn of events is not uncommon. Recantations of this kind can be adaptive denials of truth on a child's part to avoid breaking up a family, elude threatened harm, or escape guilt at implicating a loved one. But what was striking in this instance was Hannah's obvious confusion and her question, "Well, did it happen or didn't it?" If this is the best validation of fact your star witness can manage, the recantation is most likely genuine, the denial accurate.

As the threads of this case (and there were many more) unraveled, Laura's dread, which was at the center of it all, became clear. Such dread is a familiar one in divorce: the threatened loss of one's children, for a father enormous, for a mother unbearable. Laura saw Art as a better parent than herself, as a stable man with a supportive family in contrast to the chaos and instability of her own, a reality that she knew to be her legacy. Children in divorce are not infrequently sacrificed on the altar of the dread, primitive and absolute, of being alone and unloved, totally alone. Primitive fears are assuaged by primitive solutions including lies and flight when all else fails.

The Court awarded Art sole custody of the children. Hannah remained more of a skeptic than her sister about Art in particular and life in general. The biggest loss for the girls was their mother, whom they loved. They understood what their loss might mean to her. Divorce may be commonplace nowadays, but so is death, its frequency not diminishing its power.

CODA

The Ashcan School of painting in this country turned away from the Academy to the street, finding beauty in the scenes and subjects of everyday life. There is a raw freshness to its work that resembles the style an artist might use could he transform my clinical efforts to the canvas. All of the children I have seen have come to me with some variety of damage, and they have brought images and issues from the street, not the academy. All have struggled with internal or external problems not intrinsically beautiful. Yet rarely has a day gone by in this profession without some intensely beautiful experience coming my way. I think often of these lines by Yeats: "... Love has pitched his mansion in / the place of excrement; / for nothing can be sole or whole / that has not been rent." The rending matters less than gathering up the strength, in whatever way possible, to move along in life. Sharing that process with children and their families has always touched me, felt close to literature, poetry and art.

Bill Buckner, the unlucky Red Sox first-baseman who let Mookie Wilson's grounder slip between his legs to lose the 1986 World Series, became a fool to many, a hero to the wise. He tolerated public humiliation with good humor, viewing his error as part of the game. That is the heroism that matters; it will get you through life still standing. Pete Hamill writes that "...the best stories are in the loser's locker room. Winners are bores...losers are more like the rest of us...they make mistakes that they can't take back...they are imperfect when perfection is demanded and thus suffer the sometimes permanent stain of humiliation. If organized sports teach any lessons about life, the most important is about accepting defeat with grace."

My father had a favorite story he told my brother and me on repeated occasions. It involved a little Finnish boy named Sisu. I think he used it when he sensed that either of us was about to throw in the towel on some floundering effort. It usually had the desired effect in the short run and, in life, gave top billing to persistence in our hierarchy of values. Sisu was a boy whose unwillingness to quit in the face of adversity somehow, mythically, saved his nation from a terrible fate. Of the many rewards of my career in child psychiatry, the Sisu seen in many children and their families has loomed large. Like heart in an athlete, acts of will that overcome all forms of adversity provide special pleasure. The children described in this book have renewed my belief in Sisu and have proven, once again, that "the child is father to the man." My patients know that I take their lives seriously and expect them to do the same. They also know that I wish them well. Whatever part of me they have found helpful in preparing for the trip ahead I hope they pass on to others along the way. Those unable to travel, and sadly there are some, I hope are able to enjoy in peace the lives they fashion for themselves.

About the Author

Kenneth Robson was born in Chicago, Illinois and now lives and works in West Hartford, Connecticut. He attended Yale University and the University of Pennsylvania School of Medicine before devoting half a century to patient care, teaching, scholarship and public service—twenty years at the Tufts University School of Medicine and a decade as Director of the Division of Child and Adolescent Psychiatry at The Institute of Living in Hartford, Connecticut. He has authored and edited many books and papers in his field. Dr. Robson was appointed Professor of Psychiatry at the Tufts University and University of Connecticut Schools of Medicine and Clinical Professor of Psychiatry at the Yale University School of Medicine. His passions include his family, poetry, boxing, fishing, Red-tailed Hawks and the Boston Red Sox. He believes.

This book is set in Garamond Premier Pro, which had its genesis in 1988 when type-designer Robert Slimbach visited the Plantin-Moretus Museum in Antwerp, Belgium, to study its collection of Claude Garamond's metal punches and typefaces. During the mid-fifteen hundreds, Garamond—a Parisian punch-cutter—produced a refined array of book types that combined an unprecedented degree of balance and elegance, for centuries standing as the pinnacle of beauty and practicality in type-founding. Slimbach has created an entirely new interpretation based on Garamond's designs and on comparable italics cut by Robert Granjon, Garamond's contemporary.

Published by Lyre Books

West Hartford, Connecticut

Additional copies of *The Children's Hour*
are available at Amazon.com
and can be special-ordered at bookstores.
For more information, contact lyrebooks@aol.com.